KETO SEAFOOD, SOUPS AND VEGETABLES (WITH PICTURES)

SUZANNE NEWTON

KETO SEAFOOD, SOUPS AND VEGETABLES (WITH PICTURES)

182 Easy To Follow Recipes for Ketogenic Weight-Loss, Natural Hormonal Health & Metabolism Boost | Includes a 21 Day Meal Plan

First Printing, 2021

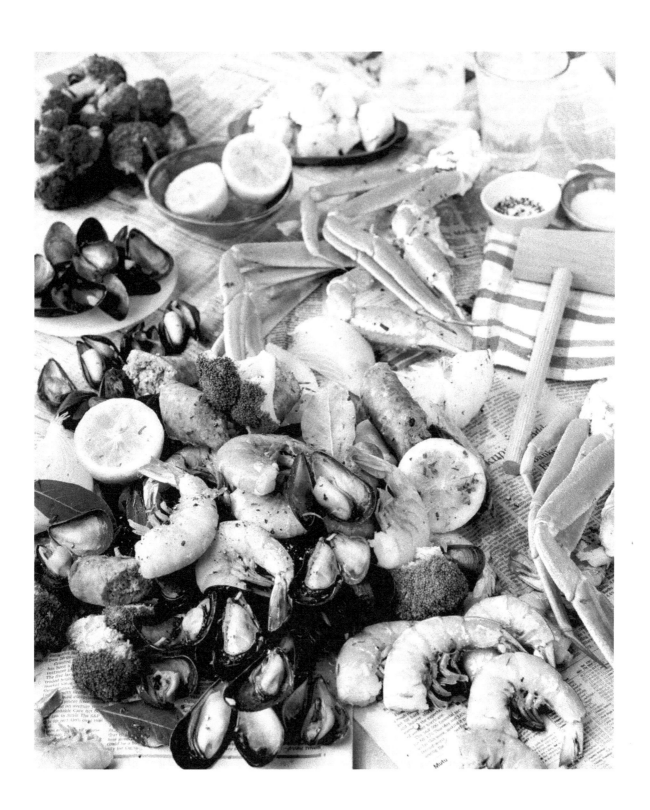

CONTENTS

CONTENTS

CONTENTS

CONTENTS

CONTENTS

CONTENTS

CONTENTS

1.   WEEK 3 MENU

	Breakfast	Lunch	Dinner	Nutritional Info
Day 15	Broccoli, Bacon & Poached Egg	Grilled Rosemary Chicken with Veggies Leftovers	Spicy Chicken & Kale Salad	1450 calories 91.88g fat 19.28g net carbs 8.4g sugars 89.73g protein
Day 16	Breakfast Egg Burrito	Spicy Chicken & Kale Salad Leftovers	Chicken Meatballs & Zoodles	1386 calories 98.37g fat 15.81g net carbs 13.24g sugars 88.56 protein
Day 17	Asparagus, Bacon & Poached Egg	Spicy Chicken & Kale Salad Leftovers	Cauli Mash & Chicken Meatballs	1165 calories 75.97g fat 21.19g net carbs 11.61g sugars 86.75g protein
Day 18	Bacon, Spinach & Eggs	Chicken Meatball Lettuce Cups	Chili Con Carne & Veggies	1318 calories 97.49g fat 19.2g net carbs 11.39g sugars 79.86g protein
Day 19	Bacon, Eggs & Asparagus	Chicken Meatball Lettuce Cups	Cauli Mash, Green Beans & Parsley Salmon	1376 calories 95.34g fat 19.19g net carbs 19.66g sugars 96.29g protein

Day 20	Chicken Meat-balls & Eggs	Chili Con Carne	Grilled Salmon, Radishes & Green Beans	1277calories 85.05g fat 21.92g net carbs 12.96g sugars 97.14g protein
Day 21	Bacon, Spinach, Egg & Avocado	Chicken Meat-balls & Arugula Salad	Chili Con Carne & Veggies + Egg	1376 calories 108.15g fat 20.34g net carbs 12.32g sugars 70.24g protein
60				

2. WEEK 3 GROCERY LIST

Baking
Blanched Almond Flour [70g]

Canned Goods
Diced Tomato Can [500 ml]
Tomato Paste [7 ml]

Condiments
Dijon Mustard [15ml]
Lemon Juice [25 ml]
Mayonnaise [40 ml]
White Vinegar [32 ml]

Dairy
Almond Milk Unsweetened [30 ml]
Egg [12]

Meat
Bacon [18 slices]
Chicken Breast [1] {285g} withskin
Ground Beef [200g]

CONTENTS

Ground Chicken [650g]

Oil
Chili Oil [1/4 tsp] or cayenne pepper
Olive Oil [120 ml]

Seafood & Fish
Salmon Fillet [2] {300g}
Spices
Black Pepper
Chili Powder
Cumin Powder
Dill
Garlic Powder
Himalayan Salt
Onion Powder
Oregano
Paprika Powder
Parlsey
Rosemary
Sage
Thyme

Vegetables
Arugula [40g]
Asparagus [10 stems]{200g}
Avocado [3 hass]
Basil Leaves [10 leaves]
Black Olives [1 tbsp]
Broccoli [2 heads]
Brown Mushrooms [5]
Carrot [1/4]
Cauliflower [1 head]{300g}
Celery [1/2 stick]
Cherry Tomatoes [8 cherries]
Garlic [7 cloves]
Green Beans [150g]
Kale [6 leaves]{120g}
Lettuce [9 leaves]
Okra [2]

Onion [3/4]
Parsley [4 stems]
Radishes [5]
Red Cabbage [1/8]
Shiitake Mushrooms [3]
Spinach [1 cup]
Tomato [2]
Zucchini [1 1/2]

3.   WEEK 3

Day 15 - Breakfast

1.   Broccoli, Bacon & Poached Egg

378 calories 26.48g fat   11.46g carbs 4.6g fiber   2.76g sugar   23.99g protein

Put the broccoli to boil in a pot of water and cook until tender. Take the broccoli out and place on a plate.

In a different pot, add some water and the white vinegar and put to simmer. Add the egg in a bowl. Swirl the water with a spatula and add the egg in the middle of the whirlpool. Cover and turn off the heat and cook the egg for 6 minutes exactly. Care- fully take it out and place over the broccoli.

Fry the bacon in a skillet until crispy. Chop it up into a few pieces and place over the broccoli. Driz- zle the sesame dressing over everything. Sprinkle the salt, pepper and pars- ley.

Ingredients (1 portion)
1 egg
140g broccoli (1/3 head)
3 slices bacon (36g cooked) 1portion sesame dressing 1tbsp white vinegar
pinch salt, pepper, parsley

2.   Grilled Rosemary Chicken withVeggies

666 calories 38.08g fat   7.76g carbs   2.2g fiber   2.38g sugar   34.86g protein

1. Reheat 1/3 of the leftovers from Day 14's dinner.   Ingredients (3 portions)

1/3 leftover from day 14's dinner.

3.   *Spicy Chicken & KaleSalad*

406 calories   27.32g fat   9.96g carbs   3.1g fiber   3.26g sugar   30.88g protein

Slice the chicken breast in half lenght ways. Sprinkle the salt, pepper, paprika, cumin, garlic and oregano over the chicken breasts. Heat the 1tsp of olive oil on a grill or use a

Ingredients (3 portions) 1chicken breast (285g)

1/4 tsp salt, black pepper,

Spicy Salad Dressing: 2 tbsp mayo

1tbsp lemon juice

bbq, and grill your chicken 4-5 minutes until

cooked through. Slice in 5-6 pieces.

paprika, cumin, garlic pow-   1tbsp olive oil

Slice lenghtways the zucchini. Heat the 1 tbsp of olive oil in a non-stick frying pan and add

der

1tsp oregano

1/2 tsp vinegar

1/2 tsp paprika powder

the zucchini slices. Sprinkle the salt and pep- 2 tsp olive oil

per over and grill on both sides until browned.

1/8 tsp salt

Boil the broccoli and okras for 2 minutes. Us-

small kale leaves (120g)

1/4 tsp garlic powder

ing a cabbage shredder, shred the red cab-

bage and thinly slice the watermelon radish.

6-7 broccoli with stem (100g)1 tsp oregano

Shred with your hands the kale.

In a small bowl, combine the salad dressing

ingredients.

On a large plate, cover with the kale, the rest of the veggies, and grilled chicken. Pour 1/3 of the spicy dressing over ONE portion.

Place the rest in some tupperwares for the

64 next 2 meals and keep the dressing separated

2 okra (20g)

100g red cabbage (1/8) 8 cherry tomatoes (65g) 4-5 radishes

1/2 zucchini (70g) 1tbsp olive oil

1/4 tsp hili oil or cay- enne pepper

4.   *Breakfast Egg Burrito*

538 calories 46.85g fat 10.35g carbs 6.9g fiber   1.96g sugar   20.7g protein

In a Japanese rectangular tamagoyaki frying pan, heat 1/2 tsp of olive oil. In a small bowl, whisk the two eggs together for 20 seconds or so. Pour half of the eggs into the pan, spread out evenly and cook on medium-low heat until the egg is cooked through. Carefully slide onto a plate. Repeat this step with the leftover egg mixture.

Fry the bacon until crispy.

Slice the avocado in a few slices. Slice the tomato in two. Chop the lettuce.

On each egg omelette, spread 1/2 tbsp of mayo. Cover with the lettuce, tomato, avocado and bacon and carefully roll up like a burrito.

Ingredients (1 portion)

eggs

1tsp olive oil 2 slices bacon 1lettuce leaf 1/2 avocado

1slice tomato 1tbsp mayo

5.   *Spicy Chicken & KaleSalad*

406 calories 27.32g fat   9.96g carbs   3.1g fiber   3.26g sugar   30.88g protein

Drizzle 1/2 of the dressing over 1/2 of the left- Ingredients (3 portions)

overs from day 15's dinner and enjoy!

Spicy Salad Dressing:

leftover from day 15's dinner leftover from day 15's

dinner.

6.   *Chicken & Herbs Meatballs*

442 calories 28.34g fat   6.47g carbs   2.2g fiber   1.64g sugar   40.12g protein

Preheat the oven to 200C/400F.

Mince the garlic, shiitake and onion.

Add the olive oil to a frying pan and fry the mush- rooms, onions and garlic until tender. Turn off heat and transfer to a bowl.

Mix all of the remaining ingredients into a large

bowl and mix until well incorporated.

Place a parchment paper over a baking tray. Make 12 large meatballs and place them on the baking tray carefully making space between each meatball. The mixture is a bit sticky, but that's fine. It'll cook perfectly in the oven.

Add to the oven and cook for 25 minutes. Take out and let cool before keeping them in the fridge.

Ingredients (6 portions)

shiitake mushrooms (60g) 1/2 white onion (90g)

2 garlic cloves 1tsp olive oil

650g ground chicken

2-3 stems chopped parsley (8g)

10 leaves chopped basil (5g)

1tsp thyme, sage

1/2 tsp onion powder, salt, pepper

1/4 tsp garlic powder

1 egg

70g blanched almond flour

7. *Chicken Meatballs & Zoodles*

423 calories 24.2g fat 17.6g carbs   12.1g fiber

Spiralize your zucchini. Cut the meatballs into 8.

Add the tomatoes, water and spices to a pot and simmer for 5-10 minutes until desired thickness. Add the meat to the tomato sauce, mix well

Add the zoodles to the sauce and cook for a minute

or so just to get them warmed up.

8.02g sugar   36.98g protein

Ingredients (1 portion)

2 chicken meatballs

zucchini

1/2 cup diced tomato can

1/2 cup water

1/4 tsp garlic powder, onion power, basil, parsley, oregano

8. Asparagus, Bacon & Poached Egg

288 calories 21.07g fat   6.65g carbs   3.15g fiber   2.64g sugar   18.21g protein

Add some water to a small pot and the white vine- gar and put to simmer. Add the egg in a bowl. Swirl the water with a spatula and add the egg inside the middle of the whirlpool. Turn off the heat and cook the egg for 6 minutes exactly. Carefully take it out.

Fry the bacon until crispy. Cut the stems off the

asparagus and fry into the bacon grease.

Place the asparagus onto a plate, cover with the bacon and poached egg and spoon the sesame dressing over. Add a bit of parlsey over everything.

Ingredients (1 portion)

6 asparagus

3 slices bacon

1 egg

1tbsp sesame dressing 1tbsp white vinegar pinch parsley

9. Spicy Chicken & KaleSalad

406 calories 27.32g fat   9.96g carbs   3.1g fiber   3.26g sugar   30.88g protein

Drizzle 1/2 of the dressing over 1/2 of the left- Ingredients (3 portions)   Spicy Salad Dressing:

overs from day 15's dinner and enjoy!

leftover from day 15's dinner leftover from day 15's

dinner.

10. Cauli Mash & ChickenMeatballs

471 calories   27.81g fat   18.45g carbs 7.46g fiber

Mince the garlic cloves.

Separate the cauliflower florets. Put some water to boil in a large pot and cover with a metal steamer. Add the cauliflower, cover, and cook for 5-7 minutes until tender. Once tender, transfer to a small bowl, add half the garlic, almond milk, garlic powder, onion powder, 1/2 tsp of salt and pepper. Using a

stick blender (or a food processor), puree the cauli-

flower until desired consistency.

Put the green beans to a boil and cook for 5-6 min- utes. Take out of the water into a frying pan along with the olive oil and add the leftover minced gar- lic. Sprinkle the 1/4 tsp of salt and pepper over and cook in the frying pan until the garlic gets crispy.

Reheat two chicken meatballs and place on a plate with half the cauliflower mash and half the green beans. Add the parsley over the cauli mash. Keep the other half for tomor- row.

5.71g sugar   37.66g protein

Ingredients (1 portion)

chicken meatballs

Ingredients (2 portions) 1small cauliflower (300g) 3 garlic cloves

100g green beans

1/4 tsp salt

2tbsp unsweetened almond milk 2 tsp olive oil

1/4 tsp garlic powder, onion pow- der

1/2 tsp salt, pepper pinch parsley

11. *Bacon, Spinach & Eggs*

354 calories 25.52g fat   2.39g carbs   0.7g fiber   0.9g sugar   27.14g protein

Fry the bacon until crispy.

Chop the spinach and add to the frying pan where the bacon was. Cook in the bacon grease until wilted. Crack the eggs open over the spinach, cover and cook for 2-3 minutes until the whites are fully cooked.

Sprinkle the salt and pepper over the eggs. Slide down onto a plate with the bacon.

Ingredients (1 portion)

slices bacon (40g cooked) 2 eggs

30g spinach

pinch salt, pepper

12. *Chicken Meatball Lettuce Cups*

599 calories 44.65g fat   17.04g carbs 9.6g fiber   3.73g sugar   36.57g protein

Dice the tomato and avocado. Cut the meatballs into four pieces. Place two lettuce leaves on top of each other.

Mix the mayo and dijon in a small bowl. Spread half on each cup.

Add half the meatballs, tomato and avocado to
each lettuce cup. Add a bit of chopped parsley over everything.
Ingredients (1 portion)
lettuce leaves
2 chicken meatballs 1/4 tomato
1/2 avocado 1/2 tbsp mayo 1/2 tbsp dijon
pinch of parsley

13. Chili Con Carne

281 calories 19.91g fat
g carbs 3.6g fiber   5.9g sugar   14.97g protein
Ingredients (3 portions)
Dice the onion, celery and carrot. Slice the mushrooms. Mince the garlic.
Add the olive oil to a large pot and add all of the
veggies. Cook for 3-4 minutes until tender. Add the ground beef and cook until browned.
Add the rest of the ingredients and mix to combine. Put on low
heat and simmer for 10-15 minutes until desired thickness.
74
1/4 small white onion (35)
1/2 celery stick (5g) 50g brown mushrooms 1/4 carrot (50g)
1garlic clove
tbsp olive oil
200g ground beef
1.5 cups diced tomato can (400g)
1/2 cup water
1tbsp chili powder
1/2 tbsp oregano, tomato paste 3/4 tsp cumin ground
1/2 tsp thyme
1/4 tsp salt, pepper
1/8 tsp cayenne pepper, garlic powder, onion powder

14. Chili Con Carne & Veggies

365 calories 27.32g fat   17.47g carbs 7.2gfiber 6.76g sugar   16.15g protein
Ingredients (1 portion)
Top 1/3 of the chili with sliced avocado and diced tomato. Enjoy!
1/3 portion chili 1/4 avocado 1slice tomato

15. Bacon, Eggs &Asparagus

370 calories 27.90g fat   8.3g carbs   5.1g fiber
Cut the stems off the asparagus. Slice the avocado. Put some water to boil in a pot and add the aspara- gus. Cook until tender.
Fry the bacon in a skillet until crispy.
Crack the egg in the bacon grease and cook it until ready.
Add everything to the plate and sprinkle some salt and pepper over everything.
2.21g sugar   22.75g protein
Ingredients (1 portion) 1/4 avocado
bacon slices
asparagus
1 egg
pinch salt and pepper

16. Chicken Meatball Lettuce Cups

599 calories 44.65g fat   17.04g carbs 9.6g fiber   3.73g sugar   36.57g protein
Dice the tomato and avocado. Cut the meatballs into four pieces. Place two lettuce leaves on top of each other.
Mix the mayo and dijon in a small bowl. Spread half
on each cup.
Add half the meatballs, tomato and avocado to
each lettuce cup. Add a bit of chopped parsley over everything.
Ingredients (1 portion)
4 lettuce leaves
2 chicken meatballs 1/4 tomato
1/2 avocado 1/2 tbsp mayo 1/2 tbsp dijon
pinch of parsley

17. *Cauli Mash, Green Beans & Parsley Salmon*

407 calories 22.79g fat   14.48g carbs 5.93g fiber   4.72g sugar   36.97g protein

Reheat the cauli mash and green beans.

Mince the parsley sprig.

Rub the salmon filet with the olive oil, salt, pepper,

and parlsey.

Carefully place in a non-stick frying pan and cook on both sides for 2-3 minutes until perfectly cooked through. Once cooked, add the lemon juice over the salmon and serve with the veggies.

Ingredients (1 portion)

cauli mash leftovers from day 17 dinner

green beans leftovers from day 17

dinner

150g salmon filet 1sprig parsley 1tsp lemon juice 1tsp olive oil pinch salt, pepper

18. *Chicken Meatballs & Eggs*

581 calories 38.34g fat   11.48g carbs 3.7g fiber   4.33g sugar   47.87g protein

Put some water to boil in a small pot and add the broccoli. Cook until tender and add to a plate with the cherry tomatoes. Reheat the chicken meatballs and add to the plate.

Heat the olive oil in a frying pan and scramble the eggs until perfectly cooked. Sprinkle some salt and pepper over.

Ingredients (1 portion)

2 chicken meatballs

eggs

broccoli (50g)

3 cherry tomatoes 1tsp olive oil pinch salt, pepper

19. Chili Con Carne

281 calories 19.91g fat 12.4g carbs   3.6g fiber   5.9g sugar   14.97g protein

1. Reheat 1/3 of the chili and enjoy!

Ingredients (1 portion)
1/3 portion chili

20. Grilled Salmon, Radishes & Green Beans

415 calories 26.8g fat 9.04g carbs   3.7g fiber   2.73g sugar   34.3g protein
Rub the salmon with the oil, dill, salt and pepper.

Carefully place in a non-stick frying pan and cook on both sides for 2-3 minutes until perfectly cooked through. Once cooked, add the lemon juice over the salmon.

Mince the garlic clove. Put the green beans to a boil and cook for 5-6 minutes. Take out of the water into a frying pan along with the olive oil and add the minced garlic. Sprinkle the salt and pepper over and cook in the frying pan until the garlic gets crispy.

Heat the olive oil in a frying pan, add the radishes and the rosemary. Cook for 4-5 minutes until crispy. Sprinkle the salt and pepper.

Serve everything together on a plate and enjoy.

Ingredients (1 portion)

150g salmon fillet

1tsp olive oil

1/4 tsp dill, salt, black pepper

1tsp lemon juice

5 radishes (85g) 1tsp olive oil 1tbsp rosemary

pinch salt, pepper, garlic powder

50g green beans 1garlic clove

2 tsp olive oil

21. Bacon, Spinach, Egg &Avocado

347 calories 31.54g fat   5.76g carbs   4.1g fiber   0.84g sugar   11.51g protein
Fry the bacon in a skillet until crispy.

Add the spinach in the same skillet and cook in the bacon grease until wilted, and then transfer to a plate. Crack the egg in the bacon grease and cook until the white is cooked.

Slice the avocado. Put everything on a plate and sprinkle some salt and pepper over everything.

Ingredients (1 portion)

3 slices bacon

1 egg

30g spinach 1/4 avocado

pinch salt, pepper

22. Chicken Meatballs & ArugulaSalad

587 calories 44.01g fat   14.45g carbs 6.6g fiber

1. Slice the avocado, tomato and chicken meatballs. Put everything on a plate and drizzle the caesar dressing over everything.

4.16g sugar   36.32g protein

Ingredients (1 portion)

2 chicken meatballs

40g arugula

1tbsp sliced black olives 1/4 avocado

1/2 tomato

1serving caesar dressing

23. Chili Con Carne & Veggies +Egg

442 calories 32.6g fat 18.03g carbs 7.2g fiber   7.32g sugar   22.41g protein

Top 1/3 of the chili with sliced avocado, diced to- mato and sliced hard boiled egg. Enjoy!

Ingredients (1 portion)

1/3 portion chili 1/4 avocado 1slice tomato 1hard boiled egg

INTRODUCTION

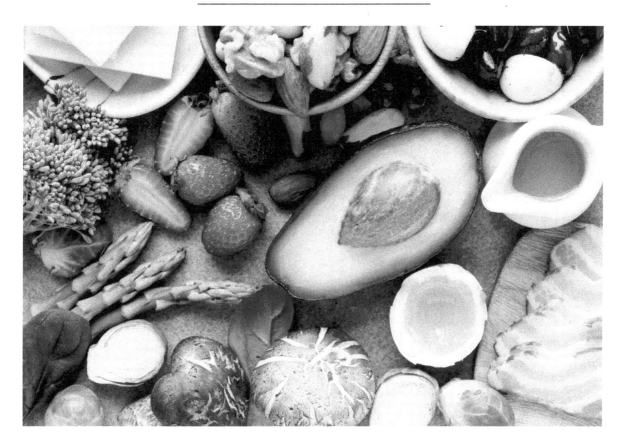

Even before we talk about how to do keto – it's important to first consider why this particular diet works. What actually happens to your body to make you lose weight?

As you probably know, the body uses food as an energy source. Everything you eat is turned into energy, so that you can get up and do whatever you need to accomplish for the day. The main energy source is sugar so what happens is that you eat something, the body breaks it down into sugar, and the sugar is processed into energy. Typically, the "sugar" is taken directly from the food you eat so if you eat just the right amount of food, then your body is fueled for the whole day. If you eat too much, then the sugar is stored in your body – hence the accumulation of fat.

But what happens if you eat less food? This is where the Ketogenic Diet comes in. You see, the process of creating sugar from food is usually faster if the food happens to be rich in carbohydrates. Bread, rice, grain, pasta – all of these are carbohydrates and they're the easiest food types to turn into energy.

So the Ketogenic Diet is all about reducing the amount of carbohydrates you eat. Does this mean you won't get the kind of energy you need for the day? Of course not! It only means that now, your body has to find other possible sources of energy. Do you know where they will be getting that energy? Your stored body fat!

So here's the situation – you are eating less carbohydrates every day. To keep you energetic, the body breaks down the stored fat and turns them into molecules called ketone bodies. The process of turning the fat into ketone bodies is called "Ketosis" and obviously – this is where the name of the Ketogenic Diet comes from. The ketone bodies take the place of glucose in keeping you energetic. As long as you keep your carbohydrates reduced, the body will keep getting its energy from your body fat.

Sounds Simple, Right?

The Ketogenic Diet is often praised for its simplicity and when you look at it properly, the process is really straightforward. The Science behind the effectivity of the diet is also well-documented, and has been proven multiple times by different medical fields. For example, an article on Diet Review by Harvard provided a lengthy discussion on how the Ketogenic Diet works and why it is so effective for those who choose to use this diet.

But Fat Is the Enemy...Or Is It?

No – fat is NOT the enemy. Unfortunately, years of bad science told us that fat is something you have to avoid – but it's actually a very helpful thing for weight loss! Even before we move forward with this book, we'll have to discuss exactly what "healthy fats" are, and why they're actually the good guys. To do this, we need to make a distinction between the different kinds of fat. You've probably heard of them before and it is a little bit confusing at first. We'll try to go through them as simply as possible:

Saturated fat. This is the kind you want to avoid. They're also called "solid fat" because each molecule is packed with hydrogen atoms. Simply put, it's the kind of fat that can easily cause a blockage in your body. It can raise cholesterol levels and lead to heart problems or a stroke. Saturated fat is something you can find in meat, dairy products, and other processed food items. Now, you're probably wondering: isn't the Ketogenic Diet packed with saturated fat? The answer is: not necessarily. You'll find later in the recipes given that the Ketogenic Diet promotes primarily unsaturated fat or healthy fat. While there are definitely many meat recipes in the list, most of these recipes contain healthy fat sources.

Unsaturated Fat. These are the ones dubbed as healthy fat. They're the kind of fat you find in avocado, nuts, and other ingredients you usually find in Keto-friendly recipes. They're known to lower blood cholesterol and actually come in two types: polyunsaturated and monounsaturated. Both are good for your body but the benefits slightly vary, depending on what you're consuming.

Polyunsaturated fat. These are perhaps the best in the list. You know about omega-3 fatty acids right? They're often suggested for people who have heart problems and are recognized as the "healthy" kind of fat. Well, they fall under the category of polyunsaturated fat and are known for reducing risks of heart disease by as much as 19 percent. This is according to a study titled: Effects on coronary heart diseases of increased poly-unsaturated fat in lieu of saturated fat: systematic review & meta-analysis of randomized controlled tests. So where do you get these polyunsaturated fats? You can get them mostly from vegetable and seed oils. These are ingredients you can almost always find in Ketogenic Recipes such as olive oil, coconut oil, and more. If you need more convincing, you should also know that omega-3 fatty acids are actually a kind of polyunsaturated fats and you will find them in deep sea fish like tuna, herring, and salmon.

WHAT IS KETO AND WHY IS SO IMPORTANT FOR YOUR HEALTH

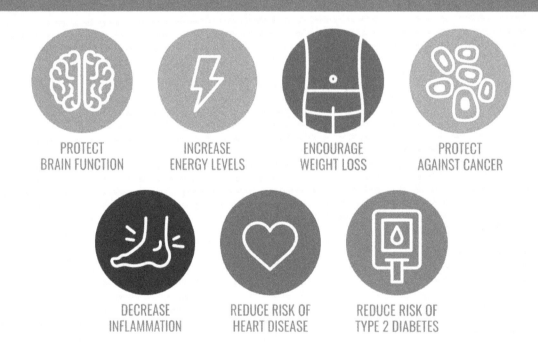

The health benefits of the Keto diet are not different for men or women, but the speed at which they are reached does differ. As mentioned, human bodies are a lot different when it comes to the ways that they are able to burn fats and lose weight. For example, by design women have at least 10% more body fat than men. No matter how fit you are, this is just an aspect of being a human that you must consider. Don't be hard on yourself if you notice that it seems like men can lose weight easier that's because they can! What women have in additional body fat, men typically have the same in muscle mass. This is why men tend to see faster external results, because that added muscle mass means that their metabolism rates are higher. That increased metabolism means that fat and energy get burned faster. When you are on Keto, though, the internal change is happening right away.

Your metabolism is unique, but it is also going to be slower than a man's by nature. Since muscle is able to burn more calories than fat, the weight just seems to fall off of men, giving them the ability to reach the opportunity for muscle growth quickly. This should not be something that holds you back from starting your Keto journey. As long as you are keeping these realistic bodily factors in mind, you won't be left wondering why it is taking you a little bit longer to start losing weight. This point will come for you, but it will take a little bit more of a process that you must be committed to following through with.

Another unique condition that a woman can experience but a man cannot be PCOS or Polycystic Ovary Syndrome; a hormonal imbalance that causes the development of cysts. These cysts can cause pain, interfere with normal reproductive function, and, in extreme and dangerous cases, burst. PCOS is actually very common among women, affecting up to 10% of the entire female population. Surprisingly, most women are not even aware that they have the condition. Around 70% of women have PCOS that is undiagnosed. This condition can cause a significant hormonal imbalance, therefore affecting your metabolism. It can also inevitably lead to weight gain, making it even harder to see results while following diet plans. In order to stay on top of your health, you must make sure that you are going to the gynecologist regularly.

Menopause is another reality that must be faced by women, especially as we age. Most women begin the process of menopause in their mid-40s. Men do not go through menopause, so they are spared from yet another condition that causes slower metabolism and weight gain. When you start menopause, it is easy to gain weight and lose muscle. Most women, once menopause begins, lose muscle at a much faster rate, and conversely gain weight, despite dieting and exercise regimens. Keto can, therefore, be the right diet plan for you. Regardless of what your body is doing naturally, via processes like menopause, your internal systems are still going to be making the switch from running on carbs to deriving energy from fats.

When the body begins to run on fats successfully, you have an automatic fuel reserving waiting to be burned. It will take some time for your body to do this, but when it does, you will actually be able to eat fewer calories and still feel just as full because your body knows to take energy from the fat that you already have. This will become automatic. It is, however, a process that requires some patience, but being aware of what is actually going on with your body can help you stay motivated while on Keto.

Because a Keto diet reduces the amount of sugar you are consuming, it naturally lowers the amount of insulin in your bloodstream. This can actually have amazing effects on any existing PCOS and fertility issues, as well as menopausal symptoms and conditions like pre-diabetes and Type 2 diabetes. Once your body adjusts to a Keto diet, you are overcoming the things that are naturally in place that can be preventing you from losing weight and getting healthy. Even if you placed your body on a strict diet, if it isn't getting rid of sugars properly, you likely aren't going to see the same results that you will when you try Keto. This is a big reason why Keto can be so beneficial for women.

You might not even realize that your hormones are not in balance until you experience a lifestyle that limits carbs and eliminates sugars. Keto is going to reset this balance for you, keeping your hormones at healthy levels. As a result of this, you will probably find yourself in a better general mood, and with much more energy to get through your days.

For people over 50, there are guidelines to follow when you start your Keto diet. As long as you are following the method properly and listening to what your body truly needs, you should have no more problems than men do while following the plan. What you will have are more obstacles to overcome, but you can do it. Remember that plenty of women successfully follow a Keto diet and see great results. Use these women as inspiration for how you anticipate your own journey to go. On the days when it seems impossible, remember what you have working against you, but more importantly what you have working for you. Your body is designed to go into ketogenesis more than it is designed to store fat by overeating carbs. Use this as a motivation to keep pushing you ahead. Keto is a valid option for you and the results will prove this, especially if you are over the age of 40.

BENEFIT OF KETO DIET FOR PEOPLE

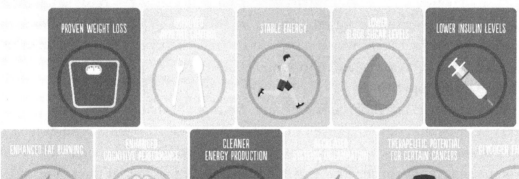

 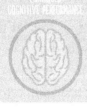 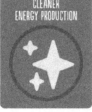  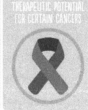 

Benefits Ketogenic Diet

Reduction of cravings and appetite

Many people gain weight simply because they cannot control their cravings and appetite for caloric foods. The ketogenic diet helps eliminate these problems, but it does not mean that you will never be hungry or want to eat. You will feel hungry but only when you have to eat. Several studies have shown that the less carbohydrates you eat, the less you eat overall. Eating healthier foods that are high in fat helps reduce your appetite, as you lose more weight faster on a low-fat diet. The reason for this is that low carbohydrate diets help lower insulin levels, as your body does not need too much insulin to convert glycogen to glucose while eliminating excess water in your body. This diet helps you reduce visceral fat. In this way, you will get a slimmer look and shape. It is the most difficult fat to lose, as it surrounds the organs as it increases. High doses can cause inflammation and insulin resistance. Coconut oil can produce an immediate source of energy as it increases ketone levels in your body.

Reduction of risk of heart disease

Triglycerides, fat molecules in your body, have close links with heart disease. They are directly proportional as the more the number of triglycerides, the higher your chances of suffering from heart disease. You can reduce the number of free triglycerides in your body by reducing the number of carbohydrates, as is in the keto diets.

Reduces chances of having high blood pressure

Weight loss and blood pressure have a close connection; thus, since you are losing weight while on the keto diet, it will affect your blood pressure.

Fights type 2 diabetes

Type two diabetes develops as a result of insulin resistance. This is a result of having huge amounts of glucose in your system, with the keto diet this is not a possibility due to the low carbohydrate intake.

Increases the production of HDL

High-density lipoprotein is referred to as good cholesterol. It is responsible for caring calories to your liver, thus can be reused. High fat and low carbohydrate diets increase the production of HDL in your body, which also reduces your chances of getting a heart disease. Low-density lipoprotein is referred to as bad cholesterol.

Suppresses your appetite

It is a strange but true effect of the keto diet. It was thought that this was a result of the production of ketones but this was proven wrong as a study taken between people on a regular balanced diet and some on the keto diet and their appetites were generally the same. It, however, helps to suppress appetite as it is it has a higher fat content than many other diets. Food stays in the stomach for longer as fat and is digested slowly, thus provides a sense of fullness. On top of that, proteins promote the secretion cholecystokinin, which is a hormone that aids in regulating appetite. It is also believed that the ketogenic diet helps to suppress your appetite by continuous blunting of appetite. There is increased appetite in the initial stages of the diet, which decreases over time.

Changes in cholesterol levels

This is kind of on the fence between good and bad. This is because the ketogenic diet involves a high fat intake which makes people wonder about the effect on blood lipids and its potential to increase chances of heart disease and strokes, among others. Several major components play a lead role in determining this, which is: LDL, HDL, and blood triglyceride levels. Heart disease correlates with high levels of LDL and cholesterol. On the other hand, high levels of HDL are seen as protection from diseases caused by cholesterol levels. The impacts of the diet on cholesterol are not properly known. Some research has shown that there is no change in cholesterol levels while others have said that there is change. If you stay in deep ketosis for a very long period of time, your blood lipids will increase, but you will have to go through some negative effects of the ketogenic diet which will be corrected when the diet is over. If a person does not remain following the diet strictly for like ten years, he/she will not experience any cholesterol problems. It is difficult to differentiate the difference between diet and weight loss in general. The effect of the ketogenic diet on cholesterol has been boiled down to if you lose fat on the ketogenic diet then your cholesterol levels will go down, and if you don't lose fat, then your cholesterol levels will go up. Strangely, women have a larger cholesterol level addition than men, while both are on a diet. As there is no absolute conclusion on the effect of the ketogenic diet on cholesterol, you are advised to have your blood lipid levels constantly checked for any bad effects. Blood lipid levels should be checked before starting the diet and about eight weeks after starting. If repeated results show a worsening of lipid levels, then you should abandon the diet or substitute saturated fats with unsaturated fats.

Risk of a Ketogenic Diet

Low energy levels

When available, the body prefers to use carbohydrates for fuel as they burn more effectively than fats. General drop-in energy level is a concern raised by many dieters due to the lack of carbohydrates. Studies have shown that it causes orthostatic hypotension which causes lightheadedness. It has come to be known that these effects can be avoided by providing enough supplemental nutrients like sodium. Many of the symptoms can be prevented by providing 5 grams of sodium per day. Most times, fatigue disappears after a few weeks or even days, if fatigue doesn't disappear, then you should add a small number of carbohydrates to the diet as long as ketosis is maintained. The diet is not recommended when caring out high-intensity workouts, weight training, or high-intensity aerobic exercise as carbohydrates are an absolute requirement but are okay for low-intensity exercise.

Effects on the brain

It causes increased use of ketones by the brain. The increased use of ketones, among other reasons, result in the treating of childhood epilepsy. As a result of the changes that occur, the concern over the side effects, including permanent brain damage and short-term memory loss, has been raised. The origin of these concerns is difficult to understand. The brain is powered by ketones in the absence of glucose. Ketones are normal energy sources and not toxic as the brain creates enzymes, during fetal growth, that helps us use them. Epileptic children, though not the perfect examples, show some insight into the effects of the diet on the brain in the long term. There is no negative effect in terms of cognitive function. There is no assurance that the diet cannot have long term dietary effects, but no information proves that there are any negative effects. Some people feel they can concentrate more when on the ketogenic diet, while others feel nothing but fatigue. This is as a result of differences in individual physiology. There are very few studies that vaguely address the point on short term memory loss. This wore off with the continuation of the study.

Kidney stones and kidney damage

As a result of the increased workload from having to filter ketones, urea, and ammonia, as well as dehydration concerns of the potential for kidney damage or passing kidney stones have been raised. The high protein nature of the ketogenic diet raises the alarms of individuals who are concerned with potential kidney damage. There is very little information that points to any negative effects of the diet on kidney function or development of kidney stones. There is a low incidence of small kidney stones in epileptic children this may be as a result of the state of deliberate dehydration that the children are put at instead of the ketosis state itself. Some short term research shows no change in kidney function or increased incidents of kidney stones either after they are off the diet or after six months on a diet. There is no long term data on the effects of ketosis to kidney function; thus, no complete conclusions can be made. People with preexisting kidney issues are the only ones who get problems from high protein intake. From an unscientific point of view, one would expect increased incidents of this to happen to athletes who consume very high protein diets, but it has not happened. This suggests that high protein intake, under normal conditions, is not harmful to the kidneys. To limit the possibility of kidney stones, it is advised to drink a lot of water to maintain hydration. For people who are predisposed to kidney stones should have their kidney function should be monitored to ensure that no complications arise if they decide to follow through with the diet.

Constipation

A common side effect of the diet is reduced bowel movements and constipation. This arises from two different causes: lack of fiber and gastrointestinal absorption of foods. First, the lack of carbs in the diet means that unless supplements are taken, fiber intake is low. Fiber is very important to our systems. High fiber intake can prevent some health conditions, including heart disease and some forms of cancer. Use some type of sugar-free fiber supplement to prevent any health problems and help you maintain regular bowel movements. The diet also reduces the volume of stool due to enhanced absorption and digestion of food; thus, fewer waste products are generated.

Fat regain

Dieting, in general, has very low long term success rates. There are some effects of getting out of a ketogenic diet like the regain of fat lost through calorific restriction alone. This is true for any diet based on calorific restriction. It is expected for weight to be regained after carb reintroduction. For people who use the weighing scale to measure their success, they may completely shun carbs as they think it is the main reason for the weight regain. You should understand that most of the initial weight gain is water and glycogen.

Immune system

There is a large variety in the immunity system response to ketogenic diets on different people. There has been some repost on reduction on some ailments such allergies and increased minor sickness susceptibility.

Optic neuropathy

This is optic nerve dysfunction. It has appeared in a few cases, but it is still existence. It was linked to the people not getting adequate amounts of calcium or vitamins supplements for about a year. All the cases were corrected by supplementation of adequate vitamin B, especially thiamine.

SOME TIPS FOR BEGINNER TO ACHIEVE KETO SUCCESS

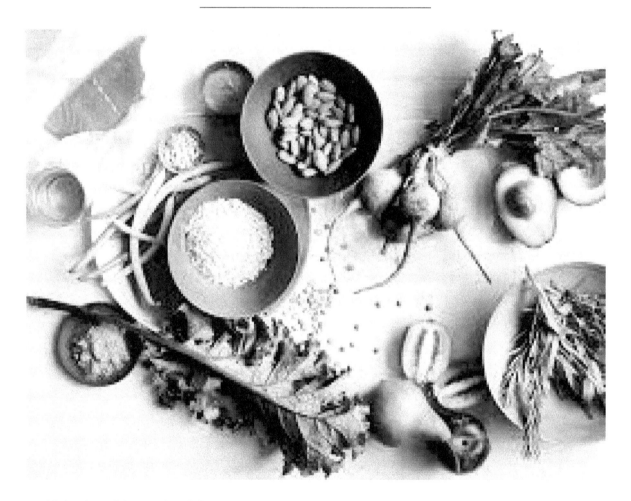

Nobody told you that life was going to be this way! But don't worry. There's still plenty of time to make amendments and take care of your health. Here are a couple of tips that will allow you to lead a healthier life in your fifties:

Start Building on Immunity

Every day, our body is exposed to free radicals and toxins from the environment. The added stress of work and family problems doesn't make it any easier for us. To combat this, it's essential that you start consuming healthy veggies that contain plenty of antioxidants and build a healthier immune system.

This helps ward off unwanted illnesses and diseases, allowing you to maintain good health.

Adding more healthy veggies to your Keto diet will help you obtain a variety of minerals, vitamins and antioxidants.

Consider Quitting Smoking

It's never too late to try to quit smoking even if you are in your fifties. Once a smoker begins to quit, the body quickly starts to heal the previous damages caused by smoking.

Once you start quitting, you'll notice how you'll be able to breathe easier, while acquiring a better sense of smell and taste. Over the period of time, eliminating the habit of smoking can greatly reduce the risks of high blood pressure, strokes and heart attack. Please note how these diseases are much more common among folks who are in the fifties and above when compared to younger folks.

Not to mention, quitting smoking will help you stay more active and enjoy better health with your friends and family.

Stay Social

We've already mentioned this before but it's worth pondering on again and again. Aging can be a daunting process and trying to get through it all on your own isn't particularly helpful. We urge you to stay in touch with friends and family or become a part of a local community club or network. Some older folks find it comforting to get an emotional support animal.

Being surrounded by people you love will give you a sense of belonging and will improve your mood. It'll also keep your mind and memory sharp as you engage in different conversations.

Health Screenings You Should Get After Your Fifties

Your fifties are considered the prime years of your life. Don't let the joy of these years be robbed away from you because of poor health. Getting simple tests done can go a long way in identifying any potential health problems that you may have. Here is a list of health screenings should get done:

Check Your Blood Pressure

Your blood pressure is a reliable indicator of your heart health. In simple words, blood pressure is a measure of how fast blood travels through the artery walls. Very high or even very low blood pressure can be a sign of an underlying problem. Once you hit your 40s, you should have your blood pressure checked more often.

EKG

The EKG reveals your heart health and activity. Short for electrocardiogram, the EKG helps identify problems in the heart. The process works by highlighting any rhythm problems that may be in the heart such as poor heart muscles, improper blood flow or any other form of abnormality. Getting an EKG is also a predictive measure for understanding the chances of a heart attack. Since people starting their fifties are at greater risk of getting a heart attack, you should get yourself checked more often.

Mammogram

Mammograms help rule out the risks of breast cancer. Women who enter their fifties should ideally get a mammogram after every ten years. However, if you have a family history, it is advisable that you get one much earlier to rule out the possibilities of cancer.

Blood Sugar Levels

If you're somebody who used to grab a fast food meal every once in a while before you switched to Keto, then you should definitely check your blood sugar levels more carefully. Blood sugar levels indicate whether or not you have diabetes. And you know how the saying goes, prevention is better than cure. It's best to clear these possibilities out of the way sooner than later.

Check for Osteoporosis

Unfortunately, as you grow older you also become susceptible to a number of bone diseases. Osteoporosis is a bone-related condition in which bones begin to lose mass, becoming frail and weak. Owing to this, seniors become more prone to fractures. This can make even the smallest of falls detrimental to your health.

Annual Physical Exam

Your insurance must be providing coverage for your annual physical exam. So, there's no reason you should not take advantage of it. This checkup helps identify the state of your health. You'll probably be surprised by how much doctors can tell from a single blood test.

Prostrate Screening Exam

Once men hit their fifties, they should be screened for prostate cancer (similar to how women should get a mammogram and pap smear). Getting a screening done becomes especially important if cancer runs in your family.

Eye Exam

As you start to age, you'll notice how your eyesight will start to deteriorate. It's quite likely that vision is not as sharp as it used to be. Ideally, you should have gotten your first eye exam during your 40s but it isn't too late. Get one as soon as possible to prevent symptoms from escalating.

Be Wary of Any Weird Moles

While skin cancer can become a problem at any age, older adults should pay closer attention to any moles or unusual skin tags in their bodies. While most cancers can be easily treated, melanoma can be particularly quite dangerous. If you have noticed any recent moles in your body that have changed in color, size or shape, make sure to visit the dermatologist.

Check Your Cholesterol Levels

Now, we've talked about this plenty of times but it's worth mentioning again. High cholesterol levels can be dangerous to your health and can be an indicator for a number of diseases, things become more complicated for conditions that don't show particular symptoms. Just to be on the safe side, your total cholesterol levels should be below 200 mg per deciliter. Your doctor will take a simple blood test and will give you a couple of guidelines with the results. In case there is something to worry about, you should make serious dietary and lifestyle changes in your life.

CHAPTER

5

WHAT DOES THE KETOGENIC DIET MEAN TO WOMEN AFTER 50?

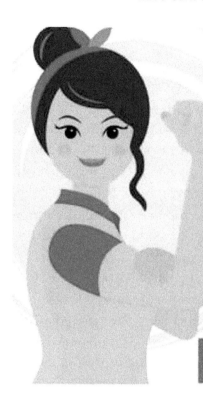

TOP 5 KETO DIET BENEFITS FOR WOMEN

ELIMINATE
BLOOD SUGAR
HIGHS AND LOWS

BALANCE
HORMONES FOR
BETTER SEX AND
FERTILITY

HELP OPTIMIZE
BRAIN
FUNCTION

GAIN BETTER OVERALL
HEALTH FROM
INCREASED NUTRIENTS

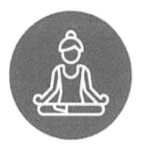

BECOME BETTER IN TUNE
WITH YOUR BODY FOR
LIFELONG WELLNESS

Why Keto for Women?

The health benefits of the Keto diet are not different for men or women, but the speed at which they are reached does differ. As mentioned, women's bodies are a lot different when it comes to the ways that they are able to burn fats and lose weight. For example, by design women have at least 10% more body fat than men. No matter how fit you are, this is just an aspect of being a woman that you must consider. Don't be hard on yourself if you notice that it seems like men can lose weight easier — that's because they can! What women have in additional body fat; men typically have the same in muscle mass. This is why men tend to see faster external results, because that added muscle mass means that their metabolism rates are higher. That increased metabolism means that fat and energy get burned faster. When you are on Keto, though, the internal change is happening right away.

Your metabolism is unique, but it is also going to be slower than a man's by nature. Since muscle is able to burn more calories than fat, the weight just seems to fall off of men, giving them the ability to reach the opportunity for muscle growth quickly. This should not be something that holds you back from starting your Keto journey. As long as you are keeping these realistic bodily factors in mind, you won't be left wondering why it is taking you a little bit longer to start losing weight. This point will come for you, but it will take a little bit more of a process that you must be committed to following through with.

Another unique condition that a woman can experience but a man cannot be PCOS or Polycystic Ovary Syndrome; a hormonal imbalance that causes the development of cysts. These cysts can cause pain, interfere with normal reproductive function, and, in extreme and dangerous cases, burst. PCOS is actually very common among women, affecting up to 10% of the entire female population. Surprisingly, most women are not even aware that they have the condition. Around 70% of women have PCOS that is undiagnosed. This condition can cause a significant hormonal imbalance, therefore affecting your metabolism. It can also inevitably lead to weight gain, making it even harder to see results while following diet plans. In order to stay on top of your health, you must make sure that you are going to the gynecologist regularly.

Menopause is another reality that must be faced by women, especially as we age. Most women begin the process of menopause in their mid-40s. Men do not go through menopause, so they are spared from yet another condition that causes slower metabolism and weight gain. When you start menopause, it is easy to gain weight and lose muscle. Most women, once menopause begins, lose muscle at a much faster rate, and conversely gain weight, despite dieting and exercise regimens. Keto can, therefore, be the right diet plan for you. Regardless of what your body is doing naturally, via processes like menopause, your internal systems are still going to be making the switch from running on carbs to deriving energy from fats.

Because a Keto diet reduces the amount of sugar you are consuming, it naturally lowers the amount of insulin in your bloodstream. This can actually have amazing effects on any existing PCOS and fertility issues, as well as menopausal symptoms and conditions like pre-diabetes and Type 2 diabetes. Once your body adjusts to a Keto diet, you are overcoming the things that are naturally in place that can be preventing you from losing weight and getting healthy. Even if you placed your body on a strict diet, if it isn't getting rid of sugars properly, you likely aren't going to see the same results that you will when you try Keto. This is a big reason why Keto can be so beneficial for women.

As we've deliberated, carbs and sugar can have a huge impact on your hormonal balance. You might not even realize that your hormones are not in balance until you experience a lifestyle that limits carbs and eliminates sugars. Keto is going to reset this balance for you, keeping your hormones at healthy levels. As a result of this, you will probably find yourself in a better general mood, and with much more energy to get through your days.

Why Keto for 40+?

As we age, we naturally look for ways to hold onto our youth and energy. It's not uncommon to think about things that promote anti-aging. Products and lifestyle changes are advertised everywhere, and they are designed to catch your attention, as you grapple with the reality of what it means to be a 40+ year-old woman in our society. Even if you aren't eating for the purposes of anti-aging yet, you have likely thought about it in terms of the way you treat your skin and hair, for example. The great thing about the Keto diet is that it supports maximum health, from the inside out; working hard to make sure that you are in the best shape that you can be in.

For instance, indigestion becomes common as you age. This happens because the body is not able to break down certain foods as well as it used to. With all of the additives and fillers, we all become used to putting our bodies through discomfort in an attempt to digest regular meals. You are probably not even aware that you are doing this to your body, but upon trying a Keto diet, you will realize how your digestion will begin to change. You will no longer feel bloated or uncomfortable after you eat. If you notice this as a common feeling, you are likely not eating food that is nutritious enough to satisfy your needs and is only resulting in excess calories.

Keto fills you up in all of the ways that you need, allowing your body to truly digest and metabolize all of the nutrients. When you eat your meals, you should not feel the need to overeat in order to overcompensate for not having enough nutrients. Anything that takes stress off of any system in your body is going to become a form of anti-aging. You will quickly find this benefit once you start your Keto journey, as it is one of the first-reported changes that most participants notice. In addition to a healthier digestive system, you will also experience more regular bathroom usage, with little to none of the problems often associated with age.

While weight loss is one of the more common desires for most 40+ women who start a diet plan, the way that the weight is lost matters. If you have ever shed a lot of weight before, you have probably experienced the adverse effects of sagging or drooping skin that you were left to deal with. Keto actually rejuvenates the elasticity in your skin. This means that you will be able to lose weight and your skin will be able to catch up. Instead of having to do copious amounts of exercise to firm up your skin, it should already be becoming firmer each day that you are on the Keto diet. This is something that a lot of participants are pleasantly surprised to find out.

Women also commonly report a natural reduction in wrinkles, and healthier skin and hair growth, in general. Many women who start the diet report that they actually notice reverse effects in their aging process. While the skin becomes healthier and more supple, it also becomes firmer. Even if you aren't presently losing weight, you will still be able to appreciate the effects that Keto brings to your skin and face. Because your internal systems are becoming healthier by the day, this tends to show on the outside in a short amount of time. You will also begin to feel healthier. While it is possible to read about the experiences of others, there is nothing like feeling this for yourself when you begin Keto.

Everyone, especially women over 40, has day-to-day tasks that are draining and require certain amounts of energy to complete. Aging can, unfortunately, take away from your energy reserve, even if you get enough sleep at night. It limits the way that you have to live your life, and this can become a very frustrating realization. Most diet plans bring about a sluggish feeling that you are simply supposed to get used to, for example. But Keto does the exact opposite. When you change your eating habits to fit the Keto guidelines, you are going to be hit with a boost of energy. Since your body is truly getting everything that it needs nutritionally, it will repay you with a sustained energy supply.

Another common complaint for women over 40 is that, seemingly overnight, your blood sugar levels are going to be more sensitive than usual. While it is important that everyone keeps an eye on these levels, it is especially important for those who are in their 50s and beyond. High blood sugar can be an indication that diabetes is on the way, but Keto can become a preventative measure, that we've already talked about. Additionally, naturally regulating elevated blood sugar levels, also reduces systemic inflammation, which is also common for women over 50. By balancing the immune system, of which inflammation is a part of, common aches and pains are reduced. Inflammation can also affect vital organs and is a precursor to cancer. Keto will support your path to an anti-inflammatory lifestyle.

Sugar is never great for us, but it turns out that sugar can become especially dangerous as we age. What is known as a "sugar sag" can occur when you get older because the excess sugar molecules will attach themselves to skin and protein in your body. This doesn't even necessarily happen because you are eating too much sugar. Average levels of sugar intake can also lead to this sagging as the sugar weakens the strength of your proteins that are supposed to hold you together. With sagging comes even more wrinkles and arterial stiffening.

If you have any anti-aging concerns, the Keto diet will likely be able to address your worries. It is a diet that works extremely hard while allowing you a fairly simple and direct guideline to follow in return. While your motivation is necessary in order to form a successful relationship with Keto, you won't need to worry about doing anything "wrong" or accidentally breaking from your diet. As long as you know how to give up your sugary foods and drinks while making sure that you are consuming the correct amount of carbs, you will be able to find your own success while on the diet.

As a woman over 50, you'll find that you will feel better, healthier and younger, by implementing the simple steps that will tune your body into processing excess fats for energy. You'll build muscle, lose fat, and look and feel younger. As we've touched on, a Keto diet helps balance your hormones, reversing and/or eliminating many common menopausal signs and symptoms.

WHAT KETO DOES TO A WOMAN'S BODY

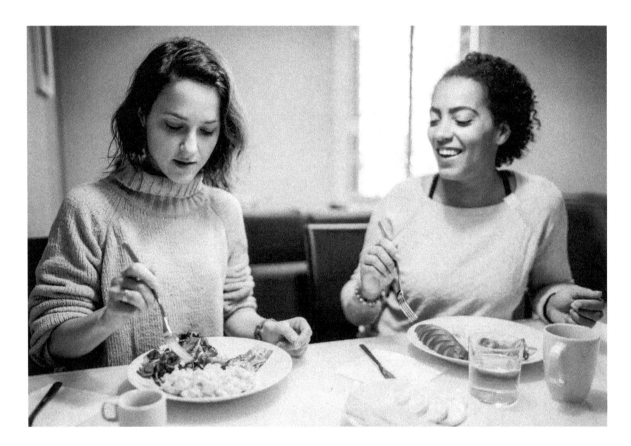

Women who are looking for a quick and effective way to shed excess weight, get high blood sugar levels under control, reduce overall inflammations, and improve physical and mental energy will do their best by following a ketogenic diet plan. But there are special considerations women must take into account when they are beginning the keto diet.

All women know it is much more difficult for women to lose weight than it is for men to lose weight. A woman will live on a starvation level diet and exercise like a triathlete and only lose five pounds. A man will stop putting dressing on his salad and will lose twenty pounds. It just is not fair. But we have the fact that we are women to blame. Women naturally have more standing between them and weight loss than men do.

The mere fact that we are women is the largest single contributor to the reason we find it difficult to lose weight. Since our bodies always think they need to be prepared for the possibility of pregnancy women will naturally have more body fat and less mass in our muscles than men will. Muscle cells burn more calories than fat cells do. So, because we are women, we will always lose weight more slowly than men will.

Being in menopause will also cause women to add more pounds to their bodies, especially in the lower half of the body. After menopause a woman's metabolism naturally slows down. Your hormones levels will decrease. These two factors alone will cause weight gain in the post-menopausal woman.

Women are a direct product of their hormones. Men also have hormones but not the ones like we have that regulate every function in our bodies. And the hormones in women will fluctuate around their everyday habits like lack of sleep, poor eating habits, and menstrual cycles. These hormones cause women to crave sweets around the time their periods occur. These cravings will wreck any diet plan. Staying true to the keto plan is challenging at this time because of the intense craving for sweets and carbs. Also having your period will often make you feel and look bloated because of the water your body holds onto during this time. And having cramps make you more likely to reach for a bag of cookies than a plate of steak and salad.

Because we are women, we may experience challenges on the keto diet that men will not face because they are men. One of these challenges is having weight loss plateau or even experiencing weight gain. This can happen because of the influence of hormones on weight loss in women. If this happens you will want to increase your consumption of good fats like ghee, butter, eggs, coconut oil, beef, avocados, and olive oil. Any food that is cooked or prepared using oil must be prepared in olive oil or avocado oil.

You can also use MCT oil. MCT stands for medium chain triglycerides. This is a form of fatty acid that is saturated and has many health benefits. MCT can help with many body functions from weight loss to improved brain function. MCTs are mostly missing from the typical American diet because we have been told that saturated fats are harmful to the body, and as a group they are. But certain saturated fats, like MCTs, are actually beneficial to the body, especially when they come from good foods like beef or coconut oil. They are easier to digest than most other saturated fats and may help improve heart and brain function and prevent obesity.

Many women on a keto diet will struggle with imbalances in their hormones. On the keto diet you do not rely on lowered calories to lose weight but on foods effect on your hormones. So, when women begin the keto diet any issues, they are already having with their hormones will be brought to attention and may cause the woman to give up before she really begins. Always remember that the keto diet is responsible for cleansing the system first so that the body can easily respond to the wonderful affects a keto diet has to offer.

Do not try to work toward the lean body that many men sport. It is best for overall function that women stay at twenty-two to twenty six percent body fat. Our hormones will function best in this range and we can't possibly function without our hormones. Women who are very lean, like gymnasts and extreme athletes, will find their hormones no longer function or function at a less than optimal rate. And remember that ideal weight may not be the right weight for you. Many women find that they perform their best when they are at their happy weight. If you find yourself fighting with yourself to lose the last few pounds you think you need to lose in order to have the perfect body then it may not be worth it. The struggle will affect your hormone function. Carefully observing the keto diet will allow time for your hormones to stabilize and regulate themselves back to their pre-obesity normal function.

Like any other diet plan the keto diet will work better if you are active. Regular exercise will allow the body to strengthen and tone muscles and will help to work off excess fat reserves. But exercise requires energy to accomplish. If you restrict your carb intake too much you might not have the energy needed to be physically able to make it all the way through the day and still be able to maintain an exercise routine. You might need to add in more carbs to your diet through the practice of carb cycling.

As a woman you know that sometimes your emotions get the better of you. This is true with your body, as you well know, and can be a major reason why women find it extremely difficult at times to lose weight the way they want to lose weight. We have been led to believe that not only can we do it all but that we must do it all. This gives many women unnecessary levels of pressure and can cause them to engage in emotional eating. Some women might have lowered feelings of self-worth and may not feel they are entitled to the benefits of the keto diet, and turning to food relieves the feelings of inadequacy that we try to hide from the world.

When you engage in the same activity for a long period of time it becomes a habit. When you reach for the bag of potato chips or the tub of ice cream whenever you are angry, upset, or depressed, then your brain will eventually tell you to reach for food whenever you feel an emotion that you don't want to deal with. Food acts as a security blanket against the world outside. It may be necessary to address any extreme emotional issues you are having before you begin the keto diet, so that you are better assured of success.

The basic act of staying on the keto diet can be very challenging for some women. Many women see beginning a new diet to lose weight as a punishment for being overweight. It may be worthwhile for you to work at changing the set of your mind if you are feeling this way. You may need to remind yourself daily that the keto diet is not a punishment but a blessing for your body. Tell yourself that you are not denying yourself certain foods because you can't eat them, but because you do not like the way those foods make your body feel. Don't watch other people eating their high carb diet and pity yourself. Instead, feel sorry for the people who have trapped themselves in a high calorie diet and are not experiencing the benefits that you are experiencing.

And for the first thirty days cut out all sweeteners, even the non-sugar ones that are allowed on the keto diet. While they may make food taste better, they also remind your brain that it needs sweet foods when it really doesn't. Cutting them out for at least thirty days will break the cycle that your body has fallen into and will cut the cravings for sweets in your diet.

It is very possible for women to be successful on the keto diet if they are prepared to follow a few simple adjustments that will make the diet look differently than your male partner might be eating but that will make you successful in the long run.

During the first one or two weeks you will need to consume extra fat than a man might need to. Doing this will have three important effects on your body. First it will cause your mitochondria to intensify their acceptance of your new way of finding energy. Mitochondria are tiny organisms that are found in cells and are responsible for using the fuel that insulin brings to the cell for fuel for the cell. Increasing your fat intake will also help make sure you are getting enough calories in your daily diet. This is important because if your body thinks you are starving it will begin to conserve calories and you will stop losing weight.

The third benefit from eating more fat, and perhaps the most important, is the psychological boost you will get from seeing that you can eat more fat and still lose weight and feel good. It will also reset your mindset that you formerly might have held against fat. For so long we have been told that low fat is the only way to lose weight. But an absence of dietary fat will lead to overeating and binge eating out of a feeling of deprivation. When you begin the diet by allowing yourself to eat a lot, or too much in your mind, fat, then you swing the pendulum around to the other side of the fat scale where it properly belongs. You teach yourself that fat can be good for you. Increasing the extra intake of fats should not last beyond the second week of the diet. Your body will improve its abilities to create and burn ketones and body fat, and then you will begin using your own body fat for fuel and you can begin to lower your reliance on dietary fat a little bit so that you will begin to lose weight.

The keto diet is naturally lower in calories if you follow the recommended levels of food intake. It is not necessary to try to restrict your intake of calories even further. All you need to do is to eat only until you are full and not one bite more. Besides losing weight the aim of the keto diet is to retrain your body on how to work properly. You will need to learn to trust your body and the signals it sends out to be able to readjust to a proper way of eating.

HOW CAN KETOGENIC DIET CAN AID WITH THE SIGN AND SYMPTOMS OF AGEING AND MENOPAUSE

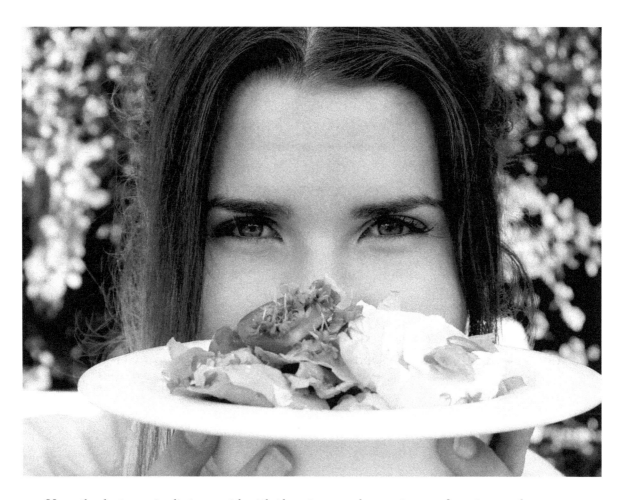

How the ketogenic diet can aid with the signs and symptoms of ageing and menopause

For ageing women, menopause will bring severe changes and challenges, but the ketogenic diet can help you switch gears effortlessly to continue enjoying a healthy and happy life. Menopause can upset hormonal levels in women, which consequently affects brainpower and cognitive abilities. Furthermore, due to less production of estrogens and progesterone, your sex drive declines, and you suffer from sleep issues and mood problems. Let's have a look at how a ketogenic diet will help solve these side effects.

Enhanced Cognitive Functions

Usually, hormone estrogen ensures continuous flow of glucose into your brain. But after menopause, the estrogen levels begin to drop dramatically, so does the amount of glucose reaching the bran. As a result, your functional brainpower will start to deteriorate. However, by following the keto diet for women over 50, the problem of glucose intake is circumvented. This results in enhanced cognitive functions and brain activity.

Hormonal Balance

Usually, women face major symptoms of menopause due to hormonal imbalances. The keto diet for women over 50 works by stabilizing these imbalances such as estrogen. This aids in experiencing fewer and bearable menopausal symptoms like hot flashes. The keto diet also balances blood sugar levels and insulin and helps in controlling insulin sensitivity.

Intensified Sex Drive

The keto diet surges the absorption of vitamin D, which is essential for enhancing sex drive. Vitamin D ensures stable levels of testosterone and other sex hormones that could become unstable due to low levels of testosterone.

Better Sleep

Glucose disturbs your blood sugar levels dramatically, which in turn leads to poor quality of sleep. Along with other menopausal symptoms, good sleep becomes a huge problem as you age. The keto diet for women over 50 not only balances blood glucose levels, but also stabilizes other hormones like cortisol, melatonin, and serotonin warranting an improved and better sleep.

Reduces inflammation

Menopause can upsurge the inflammation levels by letting potential harmful invaders in our system, which result in uncomfortable and painful symptoms. Keto diet for women over 50 uses the healthy anti-inflammatory fats to reduce inflammation and lower pain in your joints and bones.

Fuel your brain

Are you aware that your brain is composed of 60% fat or more? This infers that it needs a larger amount of fat to keep it functioning optimally. In other words, the ketones from the keto diet serve as the energy source that fuels your brain cells.

Nutrient deficiencies

Ageing women tend to have higher deficiencies in essential nutrients such as, iron deficiency which leads to brain fog and fatigue; Vitamin B12 deficiency, which lead to neurological conditions like dementia; Fats deficiency, that can lead to problems with cognition, skin, vision; and Vitamin D deficiency that not only causes cognitive impairment in older adults and increase the risk of heart disease but also contribute to the risk of developing cancer. On a keto diet, the high-quality proteins ensure adequate and excellent sources of these important nutrients.

Controlling Blood Sugar

Research has suggested a link between poor blood sugar levels and brain diseases such as Alzheimer's disease, Parkinson's disease, or Dementia. Some factors contributing to Alzheimer's disease may include:

- Enormous intake of carbohydrates, especially from fructose—which is drastically reduced in the ketogenic diet.

- Lack of nutritional fats and good cholesterol — which are copious and healthy in the keto diet

Keto diet helps control blood sugar and improve nutrition; which in turn not only improve insulin response and resistance but also protect against memory loss which is often a part of ageing.

FOODS ALLOWED IN KETO DIET

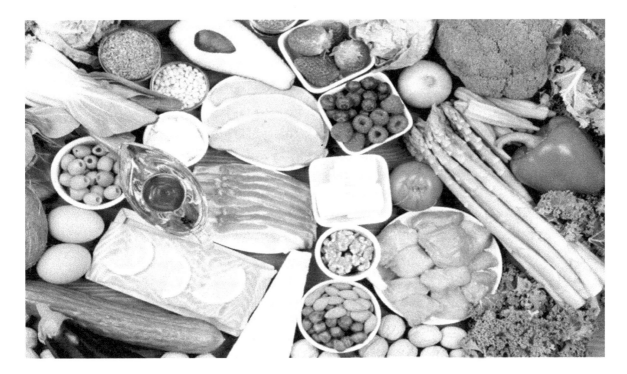

To make the most of your diet, there are prohibited foods, and others that are allowed, but in limited quantities. Here are the foods allowed in the ketogenic diet:

Food allowed in unlimited quantities

Lean or fatty meats

No matter which meat you choose, it contains no carbohydrates so that you can have fun! Pay attention to the quality of your meat, and the amount of fat. Alternate between fatty meats and lean meats!

Here are some examples of lean meats:

Beef: sirloin steak, roast beef, 5% minced steak, roast, flank steak, tenderloin, Grisons meat, tripe, kidneys

Horse: roti, steak

Pork: tenderloin, bacon, kidneys

Veal: cutlet, shank, tenderloin, sweetbread, liver

Chicken and turkey: cutlet, skinless thigh, ham

Rabbit

Here are some examples of fatty meats:

Lamb: leg, ribs, brain

Beef: minced steak 10, 15, 20%, ribs, rib steak, tongue, marrow

Pork: ribs, brain, dry ham, black pudding, white pudding, bacon, terrine, rillettes, salami, sausage, sausages, and merguez

Veal: roast, paupiette, marrow, brain, tongue, dumplings

Chicken and turkey: thigh with skin

Guinea fowl

Capon

Turkey

Goose: foie gras

Lean or fatty fish

The fish does not contain carbohydrates so that you can consume unlimited! As with meat, there are lean fish and fatty fish, pay attention to the amount of fat you eat and remember to vary your intake of fish. Oily fish have the advantage of containing a lot of good cholesterol, so it is beneficial for protection against cardiovascular disease! It will be advisable to consume fatty fish more than lean fish, to be able to manage your protein intake: if you consume lean fish, you will have a significant protein intake and little lipids, whereas with fatty fish, you will have a balanced protein and fat intake!

Here are some examples of lean fish:

- Cod
- Colin
- Sea bream
- Whiting
- Sole
- Turbot
- Limor career
- Location
- Pike
- Ray

Here are some examples of oily fish:

- Swordfish
- Salmon
- Tuna
- Trout
- Monkfish
- Herring
- Mackerel
- Cod
- Sardine

Eggs

The eggs contain no carbohydrates, so you can consume as much as you want. It is often said that eggs are full of cholesterol and that you have to limit their intake, but the more cholesterol you eat, the less your body will produce by itself! In addition, it's not just poor-quality cholesterol so that you can consume 6 per week without risk! And if you want to eat more but you are afraid for your cholesterol and I have not convinced you, remove the yellow!

Vegetables and raw vegetables

Yes, you can eat vegetables. But you have to be careful which ones: you can eat leafy vegetables (salad, spinach, kale, red cabbage, Chinese cabbage...) and flower vegetables (cauliflower, broccoli, Romanesco cabbage...) as well as avocado, cucumbers, zucchini or leeks, which do not contain many carbohydrates.

The oils

It's oil, so it's only fat, so it's unlimited to eat, but choose your oil wisely! Prefer olive oil, rapeseed, nuts, sunflower or sesame for example!

Foods authorized in moderate quantities.

The cold cuts

As you know, there is bad cholesterol in cold meats, so you will need to moderate your intake: eat it occasionally!

Fresh cheeses and plain yogurts

Consume with moderation because they contain carbohydrates.

Nuts and oilseeds

They have low levels of carbohydrates, but are rich in saturated fatty acids, that's why they should moderate their consumption. Choose almonds, hazelnuts, Brazil nuts or pecans.

Coconut (in oil, cream or milk)

It contains saturated fatty acids, that's why we limit its consumption. Cream and coconut oil contain a lot of medium chain triglycerides (MCTs), which increase the level of ketones, essential to stay in ketosis.

Berries and red fruits

They contain carbohydrates, in reasonable quantities, but you should not abuse them to avoid ketosis (blueberries, blackberries, raspberries...).

CHAPTER

9

KETO GROCERY LIST

KETO-FRIENDLY
foods list.

FOODS

- Canned cod liver oil
- Canned tuna & salmon
- Canned sardines
- Free range organic eggs
- Fermented pickles
- Kimchi & sauerkraut
- Water buffalo yogurt
- Grassfed or raw cheeses
- Assorted nut butters
- Bone Broth - Chicken, beef or bison
- Low carb granola
- Musli
- Konjac noodles, spaghetti & rice
- Kelp noodles
- Shirataki noodles
- Local grassfed & grass finished meat
- Coconut wraps

SNACKS

- Meat sticks
- Local smoked oysters
- Crackers
- Pork crisps
- Macadamia nuts
- Seaweed snacks
- Coconut chips
- Sprouted pumpkin seeds
- Sprouted almonds
- Hemp hearts & seeds
- Low carb gummy bears
- Kale chips
- Ketone bars
- Collagen bars
- Low-carb protein bars
- Sugar free chocolate bars
- Low carb chocolate bars

DRINKS

- Kevita Lemon Cayenne
- Cold brew coffee
- Instant ketogenic coffee, tea, hot chocolate
- Coffee creamer

SAUCES

- Assorted avocado oil mayos
- Assorted avocado oil dressings
- Tomato sauce
- Sugar-free BBQ sauce
- No added sugar ketchup
- Zero carb mustard
- Guacamole
- Sour cream
- Pesto
- Siracha sauce
- Miso paste

FATS

- Beef tallow
- Pork lard
- Rendered duck fat
- Grassfed butter
- Ghee
- Coconut oil
- Raw coconut butter
- Coconut milk
- Coconut cream
- MCT oil
- Emulsified MCT oil
- Biodynamic olive oil
- Red palm oil
- Pure caprylic acid

BAKING

- Almond flour
- Coconut flour
- Monk fruit sweetener
- Organic stevia
- Baking chocolate
- Gelatin
- MCT powder
- Coconut milk powder
- Sugar-free chocolate chips

SUPPLEMENTS

- Instant ketones
- Brain Octane
- Collagen & gelatin
- L-Carnitine
- Magnesium
- Berberine
- Electrolyte liquid & powder
- Bone broth protein powder

I've had people complain about the difficulty of switching their grocery list to one that's Ketogenic-friendly. The fact is that food is expensive – and most of the food you have in your fridge are probably packed full with carbohydrates. This is why if you're committing to a Ketogenic Diet, you need to do a clean sweep. That's right – everything that's packed with carbohydrates should be identified and set aside to make sure you're not eating more than you should. You can donate them to a charity before going out and buying your new Keto-friendly shopping list.

Seafood

Seafood means fish like sardines, mackerel, and wild salmon. It's also a good idea to add some shrimp, tuna, mussels, and crab into your diet. This is going to be a tad expensive but definitely worth it in the long run. What's the common denominator in all these food items? The secret is omega-3 fatty acids which is credited for lots of health benefits. You want to add food rich in omega-3 fatty acids in your diet.

Low-carb Vegetables

Not all vegetables are good for you when it comes to the Ketogenic Diet. The vegetable choices should be limited to those with low carbohydrate counts. Pack up your cart with items like spinach, eggplant, arugula, broccoli, and cauliflower. You can also put in bell peppers, cabbage, celery, kale, Brussels sprouts, mushrooms, zucchini, and fennel.

So what's in them? Well, aside from the fact that they're low-carb, these vegetable also contain loads of fiber which makes digestion easier. Of course, there's also the presence of vitamins, minerals, antioxidants, and various other nutrients that you need for day to day life. Which ones should you avoid? Steer clear of the starch-packed vegetables like carrots, turnips, and beets. As a rule, you go for the vegetables that are green and leafy.

Fruits Low in Sugar

During an episode of sugar-craving, it's usually a good idea to pick low-sugar fruit items. Believe it or not, there are lots of those in the market! Just make sure to stock up on any of these: avocado, blackberries, raspberries, strawberries, blueberries, lime, lemon, and coconut. Also note that tomatoes are fruits too so feel free to make side dishes or dips with loads of tomatoes! Keep in mind that these fruits should be eaten fresh and not out of a can. If you do eat them fresh off the can however, take a good look at the nutritional information at the back of the packaging. Avocadoes are particularly popular for those practicing the Ketogenic Diet because they contains LOTS of the good kind of fat.

Meat and Eggs

While some diets will tell you to skip the meat, the Ketogenic Diet actually encourages its consumption. Meat is packed with protein that will feed your muscles and give you a consistent source of energy through the day. It's a slow but sure burn when you eat protein as opposed to carbohydrates which are burned faster and therefore stored faster if you don't use them immediately.

But what kind of meat should you be eating? There's chicken, beef, pork, venison, turkey, and lamb. Keep in mind that quality plays a huge role here – you should be eating grass-fed organic beef or organic poultry if you want to make the most out of this food variety. The organic option lets you limit the possibility of ingesting toxins in your body due to the production process of these products. Plus, the preservation process also means there are added salt or sugar in the meat, which can throw off the whole diet.

Nuts and Seeds

Nuts and seeds you should definitely add in your cart include: chia seeds, Brazil nuts, macadamia nuts, flaxseed, walnuts, hemp seeds, pecans, sesame seeds, almonds, hazelnut, and pumpkin seeds. They also contain lots of protein and very little sugar so they're great if you have the munchies. They're the ideal snack because they're quick, easy, and will keep you full. They're high in calories though, which is why lots of people steer clear of them. As I mentioned earlier though – the Ketogenic Diet has nothing to do with calories and everything to do with the nutrient you're eating. So don't pay too much attention on the calorie count and just remember that they're a good source of fats and protein.

Dairy Products

OK – some people in their 50s already have a hard time processing dairy products, but for those who don't – you can happily add many of these to your diet. Make sure to consume sufficient amounts of cheese, plain Greek yogurt, cream butter, and cottage cheese. These dairy products are packed with calcium, protein, and the healthy kind of fat.

Oils

Nope, we're not talking about essentials oils but rather, MCT oil, coconut oil, avocado oil, nut oils, and even extra-virgin olive oil. You can start using those for your frying needs to create healthier food options. The beauty of these oils is that they add flavor to the food, making sure you don't get bored quickly with the recipes. Try picking up different types of Keto-friendly oils to add some variety to your cooking.

Coffee and Tea

The good news is that you don't have to skip coffee if you're going on a Ketogenic Diet. The bad news is that you can't go to Starbucks anymore and order their blended coffee choices. Instead, beverages would be limited to unsweetened tea or unsweetened coffee in order to keep the sugar consumption low. Opt for organic coffee and tea products to make the most out of these powerful antioxidants.

Dark Chocolate

Yes – chocolate is still on the menu, but it is limited to just dark chocolate. Technically, this means eating chocolate that is 70 percent cacao, which would make the taste a bit bitter.

Sugar Substitutes

Later in the recipes part of this book, you might be surprised at some of the ingredients required in the list. This is because while sweeteners are an important part of food preparation, you can't just use any kind of sugar in your recipe. Remember: the typical sugar is pure carbohydrate. Even if you're not eating carbohydrates, if you're dumping lots of sugar in your food – you're not really following the Ketogenic Diet principles.

So what do you do? You find sugar substitutes. The good news is that there are LOTS of those in the market. You can get rid of the old sugar and use any of these as a good substitute.

Stevia. This is perhaps the most familiar one in this list. It's a natural sweetener derived from plants and contains very few calories. Unlike your typical sugar, stevia may actually help lower the sugar levels instead of causing it to spike. Note though that it's sweeter than actual sugar so when cooking with stevia, you'll need to lower the amount used. Typically, the ratio is 200 grams of sugar per 1 teaspoon of powdered stevia.

Sucralose. It contains zero calories and zero carbohydrates. It's actually an artificial sweetener and does not metabolize – hence the complete lack of carbohydrates. Splenda is actually a sweetener derived from sucralose. Note though that you don't want to use this as a baking substitute for sugar. Its best use is for coffee, yogurt, and oatmeal sweetening. Note though that like stevia, it's also very sweet – in fact, it's actually 600 times sweeter than the typical sugar. Use sparingly.

Erythritol. It's a naturally occurring compound that interacts with the tongue's sweet taste receptors. Hence, it mimics the taste of sugar without actually being sugar. It does contain calories, but only about 5% of the calories you'll find in the typical sugar. Note though that it doesn't dissolve very well so anything prepared with this sweetener will have a gritty feeling. This can be problematic if you're using the product for baking. As for sweetness, the typical ratio is 1 1/3 cup for 1 cup of sugar.

Xylitol. Like erythritol, xylitol is a type of sugar alcohol that's commonly used in sugar-free gum. While it still contains calories, the calories are just 3 per gram. It's a sweetener that's good for diabetic patients because it doesn't raise the sugar levels or insulin in the body. The great thing about this is that you don't have to do any computations when using it for baking, cooking, or fixing a drink. The ratio of it with sugar is 1 to 1 so you can quickly make the substitution in the recipe.

What about Condiments?

Condiments are still on the table, but they won't be as tasty as you're used to. Your options include mustard, olive oil mayonnaise, oil-based salad dressings, and unsweetened ketchup. Of all these condiments, ketchup is the one with the most sugar, so make a point of looking for one with reduced sugar content. Or maybe avoid ketchup altogether and stick to mustard?

What about Snacks?

The good news is that there are packed snacks for those who don't have the time to make it themselves. Sugarless nut butters, dried seaweeds, nuts, and sugar-free jerky are all available in stores. The nuts and seeds discussed in a previous paragraph all make for excellent snack options.

What about Labels?

Let's not fool ourselves into thinking that we can cook food every single day. The fact is that there will be days when there will be purchases for the sake of convenience. There are also instances when you'll have problems finding the right ingredients for a given recipe. Hence, you'll need to find substitutes for certain ingredients without losing the "Keto friendly" vibe of the product.

So what should be done? Well, you need to learn how to read labels. Food doesn't have to be specially made to be keto-friendly, you just have to make sure that it doesn't contain any of the unfriendly nutrients or that the carbohydrate content is low enough.

CHAPTER

10

SALMON WITH GREEN BEANS

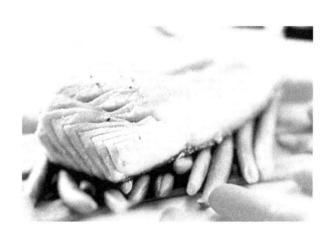

Preparation Time: 10 minutes

Cooking Time: 20 minutes

Servings: 2

Ingredients

- · 6 oz. green beans
- · 3 oz. unsalted butter
- · 2 salmon fillets
- · Seasoning:
- · ½ tsp garlic powder
- · ½ tsp salt
- · ½ tsp cracked black pepper

Directions:

1. Take a frying pan, place butter in it and when it starts to melts, add beans and salmon in fillets in it, season with garlic powder, salt, and black pepper, and cook for 8 min-

utes until salmon is cooked, turning halfway through and stirring the beans fre-quently.

2. When done, evenly divide salmon and green beans between two plates and serve.

Nutrition: 352 Calories; 29 g Fats; 19 g Protein; 3.5 g Net Carb; 1.5 g Fiber;

CHAPTER

11

SALMON SHEET PAN

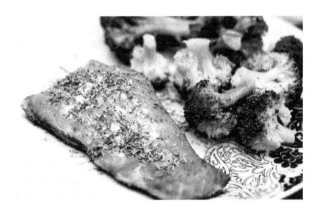

Preparation Time: 10 minutes
Cooking Time: 20 minutes
Servings: 2
Ingredients

· 2 salmon fillets
· 2 oz. cauliflower florets
· 2 oz. broccoli florets
· 1 tsp minced garlic
· 1 tbsp. chopped cilantro
· Seasoning:
· 2 tbsp. coconut oil
· 2/3 tsp salt
· ¼ tsp ground black pepper

Directions:

1. Turn on the oven, then set it to 400 degrees F, and let it preheat.

2. Place oil in a small bowl, add garlic and cilantro, stir well, and microwave for 1 minute or until the oil has melted.
3. Take a rimmed baking sheet, place cauliflower and broccoli florets in it, drizzle with 1 tbsp. of coconut oil mixture, season with 1/3 tsp salt, 1/8 tsp black pepper and bake for 10 minutes.
4. Then push the vegetables to a side, place salmon fillets in the pan, drizzle with remaining coconut oil mixture, season with remaining salt and black pepper on both sides and bake for 10 minutes until salmon is fork-tender.
5. Serve.

Nutrition: 450 Calories; 23.8 g Fats; 36.9 g Protein; 5.9 g Net Carb; 2.4 g Fiber;

FISH WITH KALE AND OLIVES

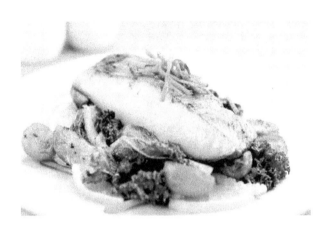

Preparation Time: 5 minutes
Cooking Time: 12 minutes;
Servings: 2
Ingredients

- 2 pacific whitening fillets
- 2 oz. chopped kale
- 3 tbsp. coconut oil
- 2 scallion, chopped
- 6 green olives
- Seasoning:
- 1/2 tsp salt
- 1/3 tsp ground black pepper
- 3 drops of liquid stevia

Directions:

1. Take a large skillet pan, place it over medium-high heat, add 4 tbsp. water, then add kale, toss and cook for 2 minutes until leaves are wilted but green.
2. When done, transfer kale to a strainer placed on a bowl and set aside until required.
3. Wipe clean the pan, add 2 tbsp. oil, and wait until it melts.
4. Season fillets with 1/3 tsp salt and ¼ tsp black pepper, place them into the pan skin-side up and cook for 4 minutes per side until fork tender.
5. Transfer fillets to a plate, add remaining oil to the pan, then add scallion and olives and cook for 1 minute.
6. Return kale into the pan, stir until mixed, cook for 1 minute until hot and then season with remaining salt and black pepper.
7. Divide kale mixture between two plates, top with cooked fillets, and then serve.

Nutrition: 454 Calories; 35.8 g Fats; 16 g Protein; 13.5 g Net Carb; 3.5 g Fiber;

CARDAMOM SALMON

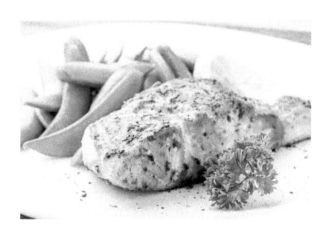

Preparation Time: 5 minutes
Cooking Time: 20 minutes
Servings: 2
Ingredients

- · 2 salmon fillets
- · ¾ tsp salt
- · 2/3 tbsp. ground cardamom
- · 1 tbsp. liquid stevia
- · 1 ½ tbsp. avocado oil

Directions:

1. Turn on the oven, then set it to 275 degrees F and let it preheat.
2. Meanwhile, prepare the sauce and for this, place oil in a small bowl, and whisk in cardamom and stevia until combined.
3. Take a baking dish, place salmon in it, brush with prepared sauce on all sides, and let it marinate for 20 minutes at room temperature.

4. Then season salmon with salt and bake for 15 to 20 minutes until thoroughly cooked.

5. When done, flake salmon with two forks and then serve.

Nutrition: 143.3 Calories; 10.7 g Fats; 11.8 g Protein; 0 g Net Carb; 0 g Fiber;

CHAPTER
14

GARLIC BUTTER SALMON

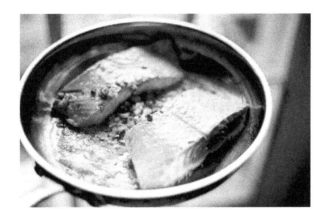

Preparation Time: 10 minutes
Cooking Time: 15 minutes
Servings: 2
Ingredients

- · 2 salmon fillets, skinless
- · 1 tsp minced garlic
- · 1 tbsp. chopped cilantro
- · 1 tbsp. unsalted butter
- · 2 tbsp. grated cheddar cheese
- · Seasoning:
- · ½ tsp salt
- · ¼ tsp ground black pepper

Directions:

1. Turn on the oven, then set it to 350 degrees F, and let it preheat.

2. Meanwhile, taking a rimmed baking sheet, grease it with oil, place salmon fillets on it, season with salt and black pepper on both sides.

3. Stir together butter, cilantro, and cheese until combined, then coat the mixture on both sides of salmon in an even layer and bake for 15 minutes until thoroughly cooked.

4. Then Turn on the broiler and continue baking the salmon for 2 minutes until the top is golden brown.

5. Serve.

Nutrition: 128 Calories; 4.5 g Fats; 41 g Protein; 1 g Net Carb; 0 g Fiber;

STIR-FRY TUNA WITH VEGETABLES

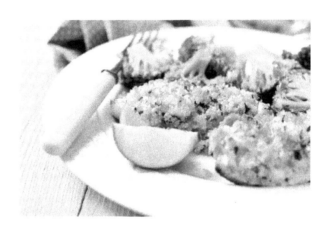

Preparation Time: 5 minutes;
Cooking Time: 15 minutes
Servings: 2
Ingredients

- 4 oz. tuna, packed in water
- 2 oz. broccoli florets
- ½ of red bell pepper, cored, sliced
- ½ tsp minced garlic
- ½ tsp sesame seeds
- Seasoning:
- 1 tbsp. avocado oil
- 2/3 tsp soy sauce
- 2/3 tsp apple cider vinegar
- 3 tbsp. water

Directions:

1. Take a skillet pan, add ½ tbsp. oil and when hot, add bell pepper and cook for 3 minutes until tender-crisp.
2. Then add broccoli floret, drizzle with water and continue cooking for 3 minutes until steamed, covering the pan.
3. Uncover the pan, cook for 2 minutes until all the liquid has evaporated, and then push bell pepper to one side of the pan.
4. Add remaining oil to the other side of the pan, add tuna and cook for 3 minutes until seared on all sides.
5. Then drizzle with soy sauce and vinegar, toss all the ingredients in the pan until mixed and sprinkle with sesame seeds.
6. Serve.

Nutrition: 99.7 Calories; 5.1 g Fats; 11 g Protein; 1.6 g Net Carb; 1 g Fiber;

CHAPTER

16

BAKED FISH WITH FETA AND TOMATO

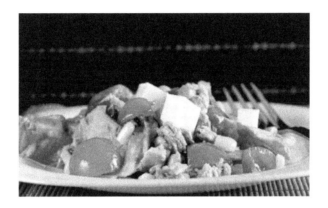

Preparation Time: 5 minutes
Cooking Time: 15 minutes;
Servings: 2
Ingredients

- · 2 pacific whitening fillets
- · 1 scallion, chopped
- · 1 Roma tomato, chopped
- · 1 tsp fresh oregano
- · 1-ounce feta cheese, crumbled
- · Seasoning:
- · 2 tbsp. avocado oil
- · 1/3 tsp salt
- · 1/4 tsp ground black pepper
- · ¼ crushed red pepper

Directions:

1. Turn on the oven, then set it to 400 degrees F and let it preheat.

2. Take a medium skillet pan, place it over medium heat, add oil and when hot, add scallion and cook for 3 minutes.
3. Add tomatoes, stir in ½ tsp oregano, 1/8 tsp salt, black pepper, red pepper, pour in ¼ cup water and bring it to simmer.
4. Sprinkle remaining salt over fillets, add to the pan, drizzle with remaining oil, and then bake for 10 to 12 minutes until fillets are fork-tender.
5. When done, top fish with remaining oregano and cheese and then serve.

Nutrition: 427.5 Calories; 29.5 g Fats; 26.7 g Protein; 8 g Net Carb; 4 g Fiber;

CHILI-GLAZED SALMON

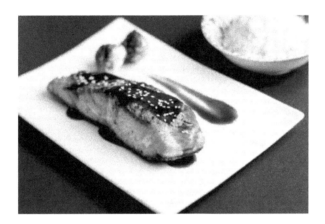

Preparation Time: 5 minutes
Cooking Time: 10 minutes
Servings: 2
Ingredients

- 2 salmon fillets
- 2 tbsp. sweet chili sauce
- 2 tsp chopped chives
- ½ tsp sesame seeds

Directions:

1. Turn on the oven, then set it to 400 degrees F and let it preheat.
2. Meanwhile, place salmon in a shallow dish, add chili sauce and chives and toss until mixed.
3. Transfer prepared salmon onto a baking sheet lined with parchment sheet, drizzle with remaining sauce and bake for 10 minutes until thoroughly cooked.
4. Garnish with sesame seeds and Serve.

Nutrition: 112.5 Calories; 5.6 g Fats; 12 g Protein; 3.4 g Net Carb; 0 g Fiber;

CREAMY TUNA, SPINACH, AND EGGS PLATES

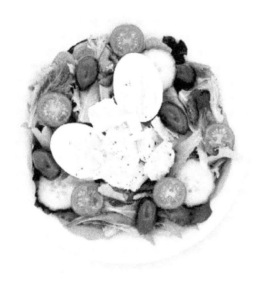

Preparation Time: 5 minutes
Cooking Time: 0 minutes;
Servings: 2
Ingredients

- · 2 oz. of spinach leaves
- · 2 oz. tuna, packed in water
- · 2 eggs, boiled
- · 4 tbsp. cream cheese, full-fat
- · Seasoning:
- · ¼ tsp salt
- · 1/8 tsp ground black pepper

Directions:

1. Take two plates and evenly distribute spinach and tuna between them.
2. Peel the eggs, cut them into half, and divide them between the plates and then season with salt and black pepper.
3. Serve with cream cheese.

Nutrition: 212 Calories; 14.1 g Fats; 18 g Protein; 1.9 g Net Carb; 1.3 g Fiber;

TUNA AND AVOCADO

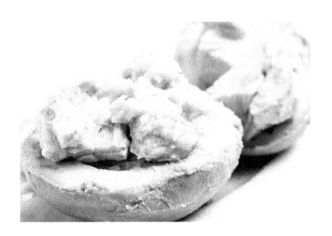

Preparation Time: 5 minutes;
Cooking Time: 0 minutes;
Servings: 2
Ingredients

- · 2 oz. tuna, packed in water
- · 1 avocado, pitted
- · 8 green olives
- · ½ cup mayonnaise, full-fat
- · Seasoning:
- · 1/3 tsp salt
- · 1/4 tsp ground black pepper

Directions:

1. Cut avocado into half, then remove the pit, scoop out the flesh and distribute between two plates.
2. Add tuna and green olives and then season with salt and black pepper.

3. Serve with mayonnaise.

Nutrition: 680 Calories; 65.6 g Fats; 10.2 g Protein; 2.2 g Net Carb; 9.7 g Fiber;

CHAPTER

20

GARLIC OREGANO FISH

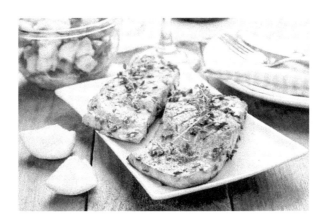

Preparation Time: 5 minutes
Cooking Time: 12 minutes;
Servings: 2
Ingredients

- · 2 pacific whitening fillets
- · 1 tsp minced garlic
- · 1 tbsp. butter, unsalted
- · 2 tsp dried oregano
- · Seasoning:
- · 1/3 tsp salt
- · 1/4 tsp ground black pepper

Directions:

1. Turn on the oven, then set it to 400 degrees F and let it preheat.
2. Meanwhile, take a small saucepan, place it over low heat, add butter and when it melts, stir in garlic and cook for 1 minute, remove the pan from heat.

3. Season fillets with salt and black pepper, and place them on a baking dish greased with oil.

4. Pour butter mixture over fillets, then sprinkle with oregano and bake for 10 to 12 minutes until thoroughly cooked.

5. Serve.

Nutrition: 199.5 Calories; 7 g Fats; 33.5 g Protein; 0.9 g Net Carb; 0.1 g Fiber;

BACON WRAPPED SALMON

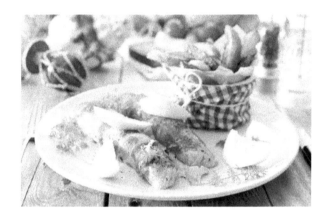

Preparation Time: 5 minutes

Cooking Time: 10 minutes

Servings: 2

Ingredients

- · 2 salmon fillets, cut into four pieces
- · 4 slices of bacon
- · 2 tsp avocado oil
- · 2 tbsp. mayonnaise
- · Seasoning:
- · ½ tsp salt
- · ½ tsp ground black pepper

Directions:

1. Turn on the oven, then set it to 375 degrees F and let it preheat.
2. Meanwhile, place a skillet pan, place it over medium-high heat, add oil and let it heat.

3. Season salmon fillets with salt and black pepper, wrap each salmon fillet with a bacon slice, then add to the pan and cook for 4 minutes, turning halfway through.
4. Then transfer skillet pan containing salmon into the oven and cook salmon for 5 minutes until thoroughly cooked.
5. Serve salmon with mayonnaise

Nutrition: 190.7 Calories; 16.5 g Fats; 10.5 g Protein; 0 g Net Carb; 0 g Fiber;

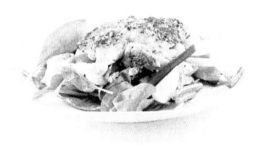

FISH AND SPINACH PLATE

Preparation Time: 10 minutes

Cooking Time: 10 minutes;

Servings: 2

Ingredients

- 2 pacific whitening fillets
- 2 oz. spinach
- ½ cup mayonnaise
- 1 tbsp. avocado oil
- 1 tbsp. unsalted butter
- Seasoning:
- 1/2 tsp salt
- 1/3 tsp ground black pepper

Directions:

1. Take a frying pan, place it over medium heat, add butter and wait until it melts.
2. Season fillets with 1/3 tsp salt and ¼ tsp black pepper, add to the pan, and cook for 5 minutes per side until golden brown and thoroughly cooked.
3. Transfer fillets to two plates, then distribute spinach among them, drizzle with oil and season with remaining salt and black pepper.

4. Serve with mayonnaise.

Nutrition: 389 Calories; 34 g Fats; 7.7 g Protein; 10.6 g Net Carb; 2 g Fiber

CHAPTER

23

FISH AND EGG PLATE

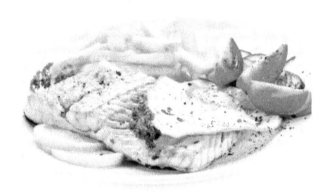

Preparation Time: 5 minutes;
Cooking Time: 10 minutes;
Servings: 2
Ingredients

- · 2 eggs
- · 1 tbsp. butter, unsalted
- · 2 pacific whitening fillets
- · ½ oz. chopped lettuce
- · 1 scallion, chopped
- · Seasoning:
- · 3 tbsp. avocado oil
- · 1/3 tsp salt
- · 1/3 tsp ground black pepper

Directions:

1. Cook the eggs and for this, take a frying pan, place it over medium heat, add butter and when it melts, crack the egg in the pan and cook for 2 to 3 minutes until fried to desired liking.
2. Transfer fried egg to a plate and then cook the remaining egg in the same manner.

3. Meanwhile, season fish fillets with ¼ tsp each of salt and black pepper.

4. When eggs have fried, sprinkle salt and black pepper on them, then add 1 tbsp. oil into the frying pan, add fillets and cook for 4 minutes per side until thoroughly cooked.

5. When done, distribute fillets to the plate, add lettuce and scallion, drizzle with remaining oil, and then serve.

HERB CRUSTED TILAPIA

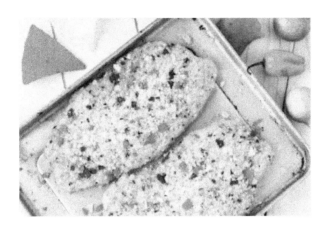

Preparation Time: 5 minutes
Cooking Time: 10 minutes;
Servings: 2
Ingredients

- 2 fillets of tilapia
- ½ tsp garlic powder
- ½ tsp Italian seasoning
- ½ tsp dried parsley
- 1/3 tsp salt
- Seasoning:
- 2 tbsp. melted butter, unsalted
- 1 tbsp. avocado oil

Directions:

1. Turn on the broiler and then let it preheat.
2. Meanwhile, take a small bowl, place melted butter in it, stir in oil and garlic powder until mixed, and then brush this mixture over tilapia fillets.

3. Stir together remaining spices and then sprinkle them generously on tilapia until well coated.
4. Place seasoned tilapia in a baking pan, place the pan under the broiler and then bake for 10 minutes until tender and golden, brushing with garlic-butter every 2 minutes.
5. Serve.

Nutrition: 520 Calories; 35 g Fats; 36.2 g Protein; 13.6 g Net Carb; 0.6 g Fiber;

SMOKED SALMON FAT BOMBS

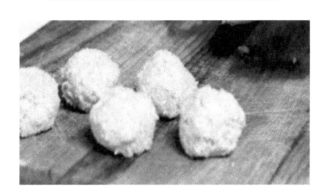

Preparation Time: 5 minutes
Cooking Time: 0 minutes;
Servings: 2
Ingredients

- · 2 tbsp. cream cheese, softened
- · 1 ounce smoked salmon
- · 2 tsp bagel seasoning

Directions:

1. Take a medium bowl, place cream cheese and salmon in it, and stir until well combined.
2. Shape the mixture into bowls, roll them into bagel seasoning and then serve.

Nutrition: 65 Calories; 4.8 g Fats; 4 g Protein; 0.5 g Net Carb; 0 g Fiber;

SHRIMP DEVILED EGGS

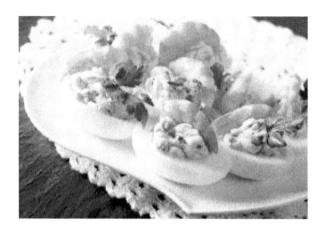

Preparation Time: 5 minutes

Cooking Time: 0 minutes;

Servings: 2

Ingredients

- 2 eggs, boiled
- 2 oz. shrimps, cooked, chopped
- ½ tsp tabasco sauce
- ½ tsp mustard paste
- 2 tbsp. mayonnaise
- Seasoning:
- 1/8 tsp salt
- 1/8 tsp ground black pepper

Directions:

1. Peel the boiled eggs, then slice in half lengthwise and transfer egg yolks to a medium bowl by using a spoon.

2. Mash the egg yolk, add remaining ingredients and stir until well combined.

3. Spoon the egg yolk mixture into egg whites, and then serve.

Nutrition: 210 Calories; 16.4 g Fats; 14 g Protein; 1 g Net Carb; 0.1 g Fiber;

TUNA MELT JALAPENO PEPPERS

Tuna Melt Jalapeno Peppers

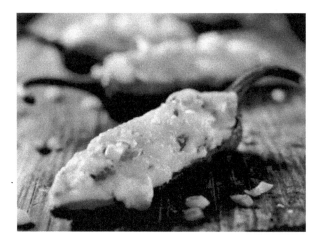

Preparation Time: 5 minutes

Cooking Time: 10 minutes;

Servings: 2

Ingredients

- · 4 jalapeno peppers
- · 1-ounce tuna, packed in water
- · 1-ounce cream cheese softened
- · 1 tbsp. grated parmesan cheese
- · 1 tbsp. grated mozzarella cheese
- · Seasoning:
- · 1 tsp chopped dill pickles
- · 1 green onion, green part sliced only

Directions:

1. Turn on the oven, then set it to 400 degrees F and let it preheat.
2. Prepare the peppers and for this, cut each pepper in half lengthwise and remove seeds and stem.
3. Take a small bowl, place tuna in it, add remaining ingredients except for cheeses, and then stir until combined.
4. Spoon tuna mixture into peppers, sprinkle cheeses on top, and then bake for 7 to 10 minutes until cheese has turned golden brown.
5. Serve.

Nutrition: 104 Calories; 6.2 g Fats; 7 g Protein; 2.1 g Net Carb; 1.1 g Fiber;

SALMON CUCUMBER ROLLS

Salmon Cucumber Rolls

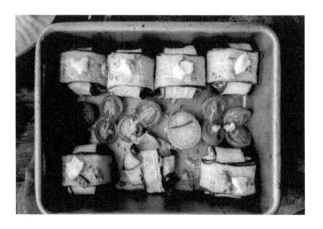

Preparation Time: 15 minutes;

Cooking Time: 0 minutes;

Servings: 2

Ingredients

- · 1 large cucumber
- · 2 oz. smoked salmon
- · 4 tbsp. mayonnaise
- · 1 tsp sesame seeds
- · Seasoning:
- · ¼ tsp salt
- · ¼ tsp ground black pepper

Directions:

1. Trim the ends of the cucumber, cut it into slices by using a vegetable peeler, and then place half of the cucumber slices in a dish.
2. Cover with paper towels, layer with remaining cucumber slices, top with paper towels, and let them refrigerate for 5 minutes.
3. Meanwhile, take a medium bowl, place salmon in it, add mayonnaise, season with salt and black pepper, and then stir until well combined.
4. Remove cucumber slices from the refrigerator, place salmon on one side of each cucumber slice, and then roll tightly.
5. Repeat with remaining cucumber, sprinkle with sesame seeds and then serve.

Nutrition: 269 Calories; 24 g Fats; 6.7 g Protein; 4 g Net Carb; 2 g Fiber;

SESAME TUNA SALAD

Sesame Tuna Salad

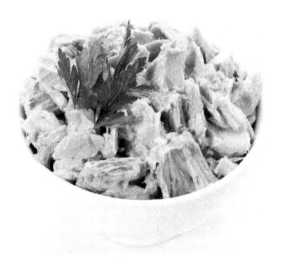

Preparation Time: 35 minutes
Cooking Time: 0 minutes;
Servings: 2
Ingredients

- 6 oz. of tuna in water
- ½ tbsp. chili-garlic paste
- ½ tbsp. black sesame seeds, toasted
- 2 tbsp. mayonnaise
- 1 tbsp. sesame oil
- Seasoning:
- 1/8 tsp red pepper flakes

Directions:

1. Take a medium bowl, all the ingredients for the salad in it except for tuna, and then stir until well combined.
2. Fold in tuna until mixed and then refrigerator for 30 minutes.
3. Serve.

Nutrition: 322 Calories; 25.4 g Fats; 17.7 g Protein; 2.6 g Net Carb; 3 g Fiber;

CHAPTER

30

BACON WRAPPED MAHI-MAHI

Bacon Wrapped Mahi-Mahi

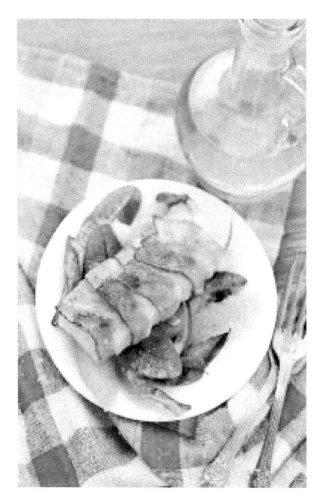

Preparation Time: 10 minutes
Cooking Time: 12 minutes;
Servings: 2
Ingredients

2 fillets of mahi-mahi

2 strips of bacon

½ of lime, zested

4 basil leaves

½ tsp salt

Seasoning:

½ tsp ground black pepper

1 tbsp. avocado oil

Directions:

1. Turn on the oven, then set it to 375 degrees F and let them preheat.
2. Meanwhile, season fillets with salt and black pepper, top each fillet with 2 basil leaves, sprinkle with lime zest, wrap with a bacon strip and secure with a toothpick if needed.
3. Take a medium skillet pan, place it over medium-high heat, add oil and when hot, place prepared fillets in it and cook for 2 minutes per side.
4. Transfer pan into the oven and bake the fish for 5 to 7 minutes until thoroughly cooked.
5. Serve.

Nutrition: 217 Calories; 11.3 g Fats; 27.1 g Protein; 1.2 g Net Carb; 0.5 g Fiber;

TUNA STUFFED AVOCADO

Tuna Stuffed Avocado

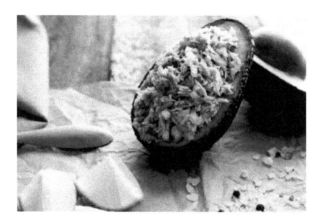

Preparation Time: 5 minutes
Cooking Time: 0 minutes;
Servings: 2
Ingredients

- 1 medium avocado
- ¼ of a lemon, juiced
- 5-ounce tuna, packed in water
- 1 green onion, chopped
- 2 slices of turkey bacon, cooked, crumbled
- Seasoning:
- ¼ tsp salt
- ¼ tsp ground black pepper

Directions:

1. Drain tuna, place it in a bowl, and then broke it into pieces with a form.

2. Add remaining ingredients, except for avocado and bacon, and stir until well combined.
3. Cut avocado into half, remove its pit and then stuff its cavity evenly with the tuna mixture.
4. Top stuffed avocados with bacon and Serve.

Nutrition: 108.5 Calories; 8 g Fats; 6 g Protein; 0.8 g Net Carb; 2.3 g Fiber;

CHEESY GARLIC BREAD WITH SMOKED SALMON

Cheesy Garlic Bread with Smoked Salmon

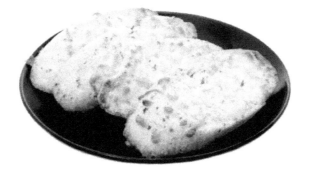

Preparation Time: 10 minutes
Cooking Time: 1 minute;
Servings: 2
Ingredients

- 4 tbsp. almond flour
- ½ tsp baking powder
- 2 tbsp. grated cheddar cheese
- 1 egg
- 2 oz. salmon, cut into thin sliced
- Seasoning:
- 1 tbsp. butter, unsalted
- ¼ tsp garlic powder
- 1/8 tsp salt
- ¼ tsp Italian seasoning

Directions:

1. Take a heatproof bowl, place all the ingredients in it except for cheese and then stir by using a fork until well combined.
2. Fold in cheese until just mixed and then microwave for 1 minute at high heat setting until thoroughly cooked, else continue cooking for another 15 to 30 seconds.
3. When done, lift out the bread, cool it for 5 minutes and then cut it into slices.
4. Top each slice with salmon and then serve straight away

Nutrition: 233 Calories; 18 g Fats; 13.8 g Protein; 1.9 g Net Carb; 1.5 g Fiber;

TUNA SALAD PICKLE BOATS

Tuna Salad Pickle Boats

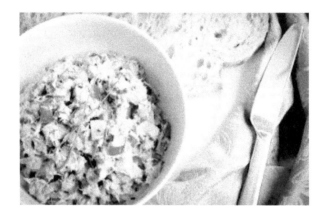

Preparation Time: 10 minutes

Cooking Time: 0 minutes;

Servings: 2

Ingredients

- 4 dill pickles
- 4 oz. of tuna, packed in water, drained
- ¼ of lime, juiced
- 4 tbsp. mayonnaise
- Seasoning:
- ¼ tsp salt
- 1/8 tsp ground black pepper
- ¼ tsp paprika
- 1 tbsp. mustard paste

Directions:

1. Prepare tuna salad and for this, take a medium bowl, place tuna in it, add lime juice, mayonnaise, salt, black pepper, paprika, and mustard and stir until mixed.
2. Cut each pickle into half lengthwise, scoop out seeds, and then fill with tuna salad.
3. Serve.

Nutrition: 308.5 Calories; 23.7 g Fats; 17 g Protein; 3.8 g Net Carb; 3.1 g Fiber;

CHAPTER

34

KETO TUNA SANDWICH

Keto Tuna Sandwich

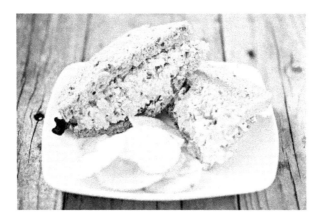

Preparation Time: 10 minutes
Cooking Time: 10 minutes;
Servings: 2
Ingredients

- · 2 oz. tuna, packed in water
- · 2 2/3 tbsp. coconut flour
- · 1 tsp baking powder
- · 2 eggs
- · 2 tbsp. mayonnaise
- · Seasoning:
- · 1/4 tsp salt
- · 1/4 tsp ground black pepper

Directions:

1. Turn on the oven, then set it to 375 degrees F and let it preheat.

2. Meanwhile, prepare the batter for this, add all the ingredients in a bowl, reserving mayonnaise, 1 egg, and 1/8 tsp salt, and then whisk until well combined.
3. Take a 4 by 4 inches heatproof baking pan, grease it with oil, pour in the prepared batter and bake 10 minutes until bread is firm.
4. Meanwhile, prepare tuna and for this, place tuna in a medium bowl, add mayonnaise, season with remaining salt and black pepper, and then stir until combined.
5. When done, let the bread cool in the pan for 5 minutes, then transfer it to a wire rack and cool for 20 minutes.
6. Slice the bread, prepare sandwiches with prepared tuna mixture, and then serve.

Nutrition: 255 Calories; 17.8 g Fats; 16.3 g Protein; 3.7 g Net Carb; 3.3 g Fiber;

CHAPTER

35

SMOKED SALMON PASTA SALAD

Smoked Salmon Pasta Salad

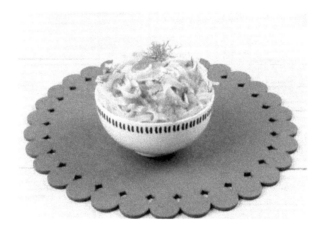

Preparation Time: 10 minutes

Cooking Time: 0 minutes;

Servings: 2

Ingredients

- 1 zucchini, spiralized into noodles
- 4 oz. smoked salmon, break into pieces
- 2 oz. cream cheese
- 2 oz. mayonnaise
- 2 oz. sour cream
- Seasoning:
- 1/3 tsp salt
- ¼ tsp ground black pepper
- ¼ tsp hot sauce

Directions:

1. Take a medium bowl, place cream cheese in it, add mayonnaise, sour cream, salt, black pepper and hot sauce and stir until well combined.
2. Add zucchini noodles, toss until well coated and then fold in salmon until just mixed.
3. Serve.

Nutrition: 458 Calories; 38.7 g Fats; 15.4 g Protein; 6.1 g Net Carb; 1.7 g Fiber;

TUNA, DILL AND SPINACH CURRY BOWL

Tuna, Dill and Spinach Curry Bowl

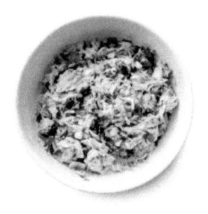

Preparation Time: 5 minutes

Cooking Time: 0 minutes;

Servings: 2

Ingredients

- 3 oz. tuna, packed in water
- 1 green onion, sliced
- 1 tbsp. diced dill pickle
- 1/3 of avocado, sliced
- 1 ounce chopped spinach
- Seasoning:
- 1 ½ tsp curry powder
- ¼ tsp of sea salt
- 5 tbsp. mayonnaise

Directions:

1. Take a medium bowl, place mayonnaise in it, and then stir in curry powder and salt.
2. Add tuna, onion, dill pickle and spinach, toss until well coated, and then top with avocado.
3. Serve.

Nutrition: 310 Calories; 28 g Fats; 12.2 g Protein; 1 g Net Carb; 0.5 g Fiber;

MAHI-MAHI WITH CHILI LIME BUTTER

Mahi-Mahi with Chili Lime Butter

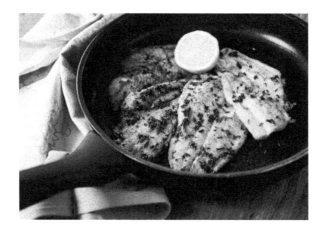

Preparation Time: 5 minutes
Cooking Time: 10 minutes;
Servings: 2
Ingredients

- 3 tbsp. coconut oil, divided
- ½ tsp red chili powder
- 2 mahi-mahi fillets
- 1 lime, zested
- Seasoning:
- 1/3 tsp salt
- ¼ tsp ground black pepper

Directions:

1. Prepare the chili-lime butter and for this, take a small bowl, add 2 tbsp. coconut oil in it and then stir in red chili powder and lime zest until combined, set aside until required.
2. Take a medium skillet pan, place it over medium-high heat, add remaining oil and wait until it melts.
3. Season fillets with salt and black pepper, add to the pan and cook for 5 minutes per side until thoroughly cooked and golden brown.
4. When done, transfer fillets to the plates, top generously with prepared chili-lime butter, and then serve.

Nutrition: 298 Calories; 18.2 g Fats; 31.5 g Protein; 0.1 g Net Carb; 0.2 g Fiber;

GINGER SESAME GLAZED SALMON

Ginger Sesame Glazed Salmon

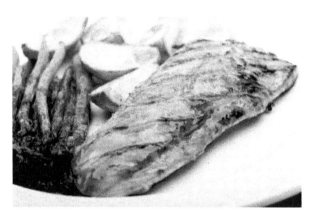

Preparation Time: 10 minutes;

Cooking Time: 15 minutes;

Servings: 2

Ingredients

- · 2 salmon fillets
- · 1 tbsp. soy sauce
- · 1 tsp sesame oil
- · 2 tsp fish sauce
- · 1 tbsp. avocado oil
- · Seasoning:
- · 1 tsp garlic powder
- · 1 tsp ginger powder
- · ½ tbsp. apple cider vinegar

Directions:

1. Prepare the marinade and for this, take a small bowl, place soy sauce in it and stir in sesame oil, fish sauce, sesame oil, avocado oil, vinegar, ginger powder and garlic powder and stir until mixed.
2. Place salmon fillets in a shallow dish, pour prepared marinate on it, toss until coated, and let it marinate for 10 minutes.
3. When ready to cook, take a griddle pan, place it over medium heat, grease it with oil, and when hot, place marinated salmon fillets on it and then grill for 5 to 7 minutes per side until done.
4. Serve.

Nutrition: 370 Calories; 23.5 g Fats; 33 g Protein; 2.5 g Net Carb; 0 g Fiber

GARLIC PARMESAN MAHI-MAHI

Garlic Parmesan Mahi-Mahi

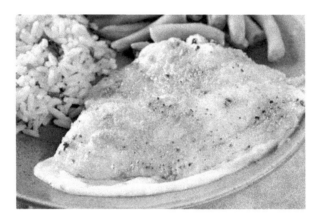

Preparation Time: 10 minutes
Cooking Time: 10 minutes;
Servings: 2
Ingredients

- · 2 fillets of mahi-mahi
- · 1 tsp minced garlic
- · 1/3 tsp dried thyme
- · 1 tbsp. avocado oil
- · 1 tbsp. grated parmesan cheese
- · Seasoning:
- · 1/3 tsp salt
- · 1/4 tsp ground black pepper

Directions:

1. Turn on the oven, set it to 425 degrees F and let it preheat.

2. Meanwhile, take a small bowl, place oil in it, add garlic, thyme, cheese and oil and stir until mixed.

3. Season fillets with salt and black pepper, then coat with prepared cheese mixture, place fillets in a baking sheet and then cook for 7 to 10 minutes until thoroughly cooked.

4. Serve.

Nutrition: 170 Calories; 7.8 g Fats; 22.3 g Protein; 0.8 g Net Carb; 0 g Fiber;

SALMON WITH LIME BUTTER SAUCE

Salmon with Lime Butter Sauce

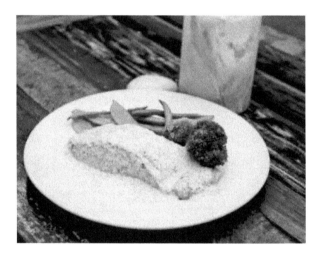

Preparation Time: 20 minutes
Cooking Time: 10 minutes;
Servings: 2
Ingredients

- 2 salmon fillets
- 1 lime, juiced, divided
- ½ tbsp. minced garlic
- 3 tbsp. butter, unsalted
- 1 tbsp. avocado oil
- Seasoning:
- 1/4 tsp salt
- 1/4 tsp ground black pepper

Directions:

1. Prepare the fillets and for this, season fillets with salt and black pepper, place them on a shallow dish, drizzle with half of the lime juice and then it marinate for 15 minutes.
2. Meanwhile, prepare the lime butter sauce and for this, take a small saucepan, place it over medium-low heat, add butter, garlic, and half of the lime juice, stir until mixed, and then bring it to a low boil, set aside until required.
3. Then take a medium skillet pan, place it over medium-high heat, add oil and when hot, place marinated salmon in it, cook for 3 minutes per side and then transfer to a plate.
4. Top each salmon with prepared lime butter sauce and then serve.

Nutrition: 192 Calories; 18 g Fats; 6 g Protein; 4 g Net Carb; 0 g Fiber;

MUSHROOM WITH SALMON

Mushroom with Salmon

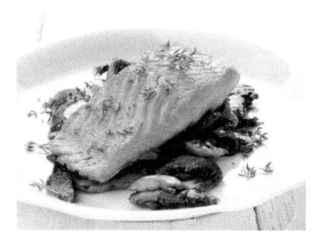

Preparation Time: 5 minutes
Cooking Time: 15 minutes;
Servings: 2
Ingredients

- · 2 salmon fillets
- · 2 oz. sliced mushrooms
- · 1 tbsp. avocado oil
- · 3 tbsp. butter, unsalted
- · ¼ cup of water
- · Seasoning:
- · 3/4 tsp salt
- · 1/2 tsp ground black pepper
- · ¼ tsp paprika

Directions:

1. Take a medium skillet pan, place it over medium heat, add oil and wait until it gets hot.
2. Season salmon with ½ tsp salt and ¼ tsp black pepper, add them to the pan and cook for 3 minutes per side until brown, set aside until done.
3. Add 2 tbsp. butter into the pan and when it melts, add mushrooms, season with paprika and remaining salt and black pepper, and cook for 3 minutes until sauté.
4. Pour in water, stir well, then add remaining butter and when it melts, return pork chops into the pan and simmer for 3 minutes until cooked.
5. Serve.

Nutrition: 420 Calories; 34.2 g Fats; 25 g Protein; 1.8 g Net Carb; 0.3 g Fiber;

BLACKENED FISH WITH ZUCCHINI NOODLES

Blackened Fish with Zucchini Noodles

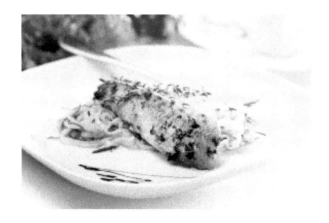

Preparation Time: 10 minutes;

Cooking Time: 12 minutes;

Servings: 2

Ingredients

- · 1 large zucchini
- · 2 fillets of mahi-mahi
- · 1 tsp Cajun seasoning
- · 2 tbsp. butter, unsalted
- · 1 tbsp. avocado oil
- · Seasoning:
- · ½ tsp garlic powder
- · 2/3 tsp salt
- · ½ tsp ground black pepper

Directions:

1. Spiralized zucchini into noodles, place them into a colander, sprinkle with 1/3 tsp salt, toss until mixed and set aside until required.
2. Meanwhile, prepare fish and for this, season fillets with remaining salt and ¾ tsp Cajun seasoning.
3. Take a medium skillet pan, place it over medium heat, add butter and when it melts, add prepared fillets, switch heat to medium-high level and cook for 3 to 4 minutes per side until cooked and nicely browned.
4. Transfer fillets to a plate and then reserve the pan for zucchini noodles.
5. Squeeze moisture from the noodles, add them to the skillet pan, add oil, toss until mixed, season with remaining Cajun seasoning and cook for 2 to 3 minutes until noodles have turned soft.
6. Sprinkle with garlic powder, remove the pan from heat and distribute noodles between two plates.
7. Top noodles with a fillet and then serve.

Nutrition: 350 Calories; 25 g Fats; 27.1 g Protein; 2.8 g Net Carb; 1.6 g Fiber;

ZUCCHINI NOODLES IN CREAMY SALMON SAUCE

Zucchini Noodles in Creamy Salmon Sauce

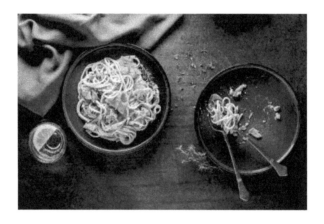

Preparation Time: 5 minutes;

Cooking Time: 7 minutes;

Servings: 2

Ingredients

- 3 oz. smoked salmon
- 1 zucchini, spiralized into noodles
- 1 tbsp. chopped basil
- 2 oz. whipping cream
- 2 oz. cream cheese, softened
- Seasoning:
- 1/3 tsp salt
- 1/3 tsp ground black pepper
- 1 tbsp. avocado oil

Directions:

1. Cut zucchini into noodles, place them into a colander, sprinkle with some salt, toss until well coated and set aside for 10 minutes.
2. Meanwhile, take a small saucepan, place it over medium-low heat, add whipped cream in it, add cream cheese, stir until mixed, bring it to a simmer, and cook for 2 minutes or more until smooth.
3. Then switch heat to low heat, add basil into the pan, cut salmon into thin slices, add to the pan, season with ¼ tsp of each salt and black pepper and cook for 1 minute until hot, set aside until required.
4. Take a medium skillet pan, place it over medium-high heat, add oil and when hot, add zucchini noodles and cook for 1 to 2 minutes until fried.
5. Season zucchini with remaining salt and black pepper and then distribute zucchini between two plates.
6. Top zucchini noodles with salmon sauce and then serve.

Nutrition: 271 Calories; 22 g Fats; 13.5 g Protein; 4.5 g Net Carb; 1.5 g Fiber;

TUNA SALAD CUCUMBER BOATS

Tuna Salad Cucumber Boats

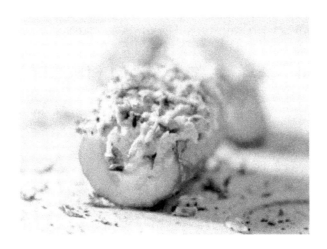

Preparation Time: 10 minutes
Cooking Time: 0 minutes;
Servings: 2
Ingredients

· 1 cucumber
· 2 oz. tuna, packed in water
· 1 green onion, sliced
· 2 1/2 tbsp. mayonnaise
· 1 tsp mustard paste
· Seasoning:
· ¼ tsp salt
· 1/8 tsp ground black pepper

Directions:

1. Prepare salad and for this, place tuna in a bowl, add onion, mayonnaise and mustard, then add salt and black pepper and stir until combined.
2. Cut cucumber from the middle lengthwise, then scrape out the inside by using a spoon and fill the space with tuna salad.
3. Serve.

Nutrition: 190 Calories; 14.2 g Fats; 8.8 g Protein; 3.6 g Net Carb; 2 g Fiber;

SOUP AND STEW

·

Chicken Enchilada Soup

Preparation Time: 10 minutes
Cooking Time: 45 minutes
Servings: 4
Ingredients:

- ½ c. fresh cilantro, chopped
- 1 ¼ tsp. chili powder
- 1 c. fresh tomatoes, diced
- 1 med. yellow onion, diced
- 1 sm. red bell pepper, diced
- 1 tbsp. cumin, ground
- 1 tbsp. extra virgin olive oil
- 1 tbsp. lime juice, fresh
- 1 tsp. dried oregano
- 2 cloves garlic, minced
- 2 lg. stalks celery, diced
- 4 c. chicken broth
- 8 oz. chicken thighs, boneless & skinless, shredded
- 8 oz. cream cheese, softened

Direction:

1. In a pot over medium heat, warm olive oil.
2. Once hot, add celery, red pepper, onion, and garlic. Cook for about 3 minutes or until shiny.
3. Stir the tomatoes into the pot and let cook for another 2 minutes.
4. Add seasonings to the pot, stir in chicken broth and bring to a boil.

5. Once boiling, drop the heat down to low and allow to simmer for 20 minutes.

6. Once simmered, add the cream cheese and allow the soup to return to a boil. *

7. Drop the heat once again and allow to simmer for another 20 minutes.

8. Stir the shredded chicken into the soup along with the lime juice and the cilantro.

9. Spoon into bowls and serve hot!

Nutrition:

Calories: 420

Carbohydrates: 9 grams

Fat: 29.5 grams

Protein: 27 grams

BUFFALO CHICKEN SOUP

Preparation Time: 20 minutes
Cooking Time: 20 minutes
Servings: 4
Ingredients:

- 4 med. stalks celery, diced
- 2 med. carrots, diced
- 4 chicken breasts, boneless & skinless
- 6 tbsp. butter
- 1 qt. chicken broth
- 2 oz. cream cheese
- ½ c. heavy cream
- ½ c. buffalo sauce 1 tsp. sea salt
- ½ tsp. thyme, dried
- For garnish:
- Sour cream
- Green onions, thinly sliced
- Bleu cheese crumbles

Direction:

1. Set a large pot to warm over medium heat with the olive oil in it.
2. Cook celery and carrot until shiny and tender. Add chicken breasts to the pot and cover. Allow to cook about five to six minutes per side. Once the chicken has cooked and formed some caramelization on each side, remove it from the pot.
3. Shred the chicken breasts and set aside. Pour the chicken broth into the pot with the carrots and celery, then stir in the cream, butter, and cream cheese. * Bring the pot to

a boil, then add chicken back to the pot. Stir buffalo sauce into the mix and combine completely. Feel free to increase or decrease as desired.

4. Add seasonings, stir, and drop the heat to low. Allow the soup to simmer for 15 to 20 minutes, or until all the flavors have fully combined. Serve hot with a garnish of sour cream, bleu cheese crumbles, and sliced green onion!

Nutrition:

Calories: 563

Carbohydrates: 4 grams

Fat: 32.5 grams

Protein: 57 grams

THE SALSA

Preparation Time: 20 minutes
Cooking Time: 40 minutes
Servings: 1
Ingredients

- One small tomato
- One Thai chili, thinly sliced.
- One teaspoon of caper, fine cut
- Parsley - 2 teaspoons fine cut
- 1/4 of a lemon's juice

Directions

1. Remove the eye from the tomato to make the salsa and slice it finely, ensuring that the fluid remains in as much as possible. Combine chile, capers, lemon juice and parsley. You might mix it all in, but the end product is a little different.
2. Oven to 220 degrees Celsius (425 ° F), in one teaspoon, marinate the chicken breast with a little oil and lemon juice. Leave for five to ten minutes.
3. Then add the marinated chicken and cook on either side for about a minute, until pale golden, transfer to the oven (on a baking tray, if your pan is not ovenproof), 8 to 10 minutes or until cooked. Remove from the oven, cover with tape, and wait until eaten for five minutes.
4. Cook the kale for 5 minutes in a steamer in the meantime, add a little butter, fry the red onions and the ginger and then mix in the fluffy but not browned mix.
5. Cook the buckwheat with the remaining teaspoon of turmeric according to the package instructions. Eat rice, tomatoes and salsa. Eat together.

Nutrition:

Calories: 104,

Sodium: 33 mg,

Dietary Fibre: 1.6 g,

Total Fat: 4.3 g,

Total Carbs: 15.3 g,

Protein: 1.3 g.

RAS-EL-HANOUT HOT SAUCE

Preparation Time: 10 minutes
Cooking Time: 10 minutes
Servings: 2
Ingredients:

- Olive oil
- Lemon slices (juice)
- Teaspoon honey
- 1½ teaspoons Ras el Hanout
- 1/2 red peppers, prepare:

Directions:

1. Remove the seeds from the pepper.
2. Chopped peppers.
3. Put pepper in a bowl filled with lemon juice, honey and Ras-ElHanout and mix.
4. Then add olive oil drop by drop while continuing to mix. Sweet and Sour Pot:

Nutrition:
Calories: 1495,
Sodium: 33 mg,
Dietary Fibre: 1.6 g,
Total Fat: 3.1 g,
Total Carbs: 16.5 g,
Protein: 1.3 g.

TERIYAKI SAUCE

Preparation Time: 10 minutes
Cooking Time: 30 minutes
Servings: 1
Ingredients

- 7fl oz. soy sauce
- 7fl oz. pineapple juice
- 1 teaspoon red wine vinegar
- 1-inch chunk of fresh ginger root, peeled and chopped
- 2 cloves of garlic

Directions

1. Place the ingredients into a saucepan, bring them to the boil, reduce the heat and simmer for 10 minutes. Let it cool then remove the garlic and ginger. Store it in a container in the fridge until ready to use. Use as a marinade for meat, fish and tofu dishes.

Nutrition:
Calories: 267,
Sodium: 33 mg,
Dietary Fibre: 1.2 g,
Total Fat: 4.3 g,
Total Carbs: 16.2 g,
Protein: 1.3 g.

GARLIC VINAIGRETTE

Preparation Time: 10 minutes
Cooking Time: 30 minutes
Servings: 1
Ingredients

- 1 clove garlic, crushed
- 4 tablespoons olive oil
- 1 tablespoon lemon juice
- Freshly ground black pepper

Directions

1. Simply mix all of the ingredients together. It can either be stored or used straight away.

Nutrition:
Calories: 104,
Sodium: 35 mg,
Dietary Fibre: 1.3 g,
Total Fat: 3.1 g,
Total Carbs: 16.2 g,
Protein: 1.3 g.

LEMON CAPER PESTO

Preparation Time: 10 minutes
Cooking Time: 10 minutes
Servings: 1
Ingredients

· 6 tablespoons fresh parsley leaves
· 3 cloves of garlic
· 2 tablespoons capers
· 2oz cashew nuts
· 2 tablespoons olive oil
· 1 tablespoon lemon juice

Directions

1. Place all of the ingredients into a food processor and blitz until smooth. Add a little extra oil if necessary. Serve with pasta, vegetables or meat dishes.

Nutrition:
Calories: 250,
Sodium: 32 mg,
Dietary Fibre: 1.6 g,
Total Fat: 4.1 g,
Total Carbs: 16.4 g,
Protein: 1.5 g.

PARSLEY PESTO

Preparation Time: 10 minutes

Cooking Time: 10 minutes

Servings: 1

Ingredients

- 3oz Parmesan cheese, finely grated
- 2oz pine nuts
- 6 tablespoons fresh parsley leaves, chopped
- 2 cloves of garlic
- 2 tablespoons olive oil

Direction

1. Put all of the ingredients into a food processor or blend until you have a smooth paste.

Nutrition:

Calories: 104,

Sodium: 32 mg,

Dietary Fibre: 1.6 g,

Total Fat: 4.3 g,

Total Carbs: 16.2 g,

Protein: 1.3 g.

SLOW COOKER TACO SOUP

Preparation Time: 10 minutes
Cooking Time: 2 hours
Servings: 8
Ingredients:

- ¼ c. sour cream
- ½ c. cheddar cheese, shredded
- 2 c. diced tomatoes
- 2 lbs. ground beef
- 3 tbsp. taco seasoning*
- 4 c. chicken broth
- 8 oz. cream cheese, cubed**

Direction:

1. Heat a medium saucepan over medium heat and brown the beef.
2. Drain the fat from the beef and then place it into the slow cooker.
3. Add the cream cheese cubes, taco seasoning, and diced tomatoes into the slow cooker.
4. Add the chicken broth, cover and leave to cook on high for two hours.
5. Once the timer is up, stir all the ingredients and spoon the soup into bowls.
6. Serve hot with sour cream and shredded cheese on top!
7. *Check the label! Make sure that the taco seasoning you buy doesn't contain hidden sugars or starches.
8. **Cream cheese is easier to cut when it's very cold and if you carefully spread a little bit of olive oil on the blade of the knife!

Nutrition:

Calories: 505
Carbohydrates: 8.5 grams
Fat: 31.5 grams
Protein: 43.5 grams

WALNUT VINAIGRETTE

Preparation Time: 10 minutes
Cooking Time: 10 minutes
Servings: 1
Ingredients

- 1 clove garlic, finely chopped
- 6 tablespoons olive oil
- 3 tablespoons red wine vinegar
- 1 tablespoon walnut oil
- Sea salt
- Freshly ground black pepper

Directions

1. Combine all of the ingredients in a bowl or container and season with salt and pepper. Use immediately or store in the fridge.

Nutrition:
Calories: 109,
Sodium: 33 mg,
Dietary Fibre: 1.6 g,
Total Fat: 4.3 g,
Total Carbs: 16.4 g,
Protein: 1.6 g.

TURMERIC & LEMON DRESSING

Preparation Time: 10 minutes

Cooking Time: 30 minutes

Servings: 1

Ingredients

- · 1 teaspoon turmeric
- · 4 tablespoons olive oil
- · Juice of 1 lemon

Directions

1. Combine all the ingredients in bowl and serve with salads. Eat straight away.

Nutrition:

Calories: 125,

Sodium: 32 mg,

Dietary Fibre: 1.6 g,

Total Fat: 3.3 g,

Total Carbs: 16.3 g,

Protein: 1.5 g.

WALNUT & MINT PESTO

Preparation Time: 10 minutes
Cooking Time: 10 minutes
Servings: 1
Ingredients

- 6 tablespoons fresh mint leaves
- 2oz walnuts
- 2 cloves of garlic
- 3½oz Parmesan cheese
- 1 tablespoon lemon juice

Direction

1. Put all the ingredients into a food processor and blend until it becomes a smooth paste.

Nutrition:
Calories: 99,
Sodium: 33 mg,
Dietary Fibre: 1.6 g,
Total Fat: 4.4 g,
Total Carbs: 16.4 g,
Protein: 1.6 g.

WEDDING SOUP

Preparation Time: 5 minutes
Cooking Time: 10 minutes
Servings: 4
Ingredients:

- ½ c. almond flour
- ½ c. parmesan cheese, grated
- ½ sm. yellow onion, diced
- 1 lb. ground beef
- 1 lg. egg, beaten
- 1 tsp. Italian seasoning
- 1 tsp. oregano, fresh & chopped
- 1 tsp. thyme, fresh & chopped
- 2 c. baby leaf spinach, fresh
- 2 c. cauliflower, riced
- 2 med. stalks celery, diced
- 2 tbsp. extra virgin olive oil
- 3 cloves garlic, minced
- 6 c. chicken broth
- Sea salt & pepper to taste

Direction:

1. In a large mixing bowl, combine almond flour, parmesan cheese, ground beef, egg, salt, pepper, and Italian seasoning. Mix thoroughly by band
2. Shape the meat mixture into one-inch meatballs, cover, and refrigerate until ready to cook.
3. In a large saucepan over medium heat, warm the olive oil.

4. Once the oil is hot, stir the celery and onion into the pan and season to taste with salt and pepper.
5. Stirring often, bring the onion and celery to a lightly cooked state, about six or seven minutes.
6. Add the garlic to the pan, stir to combine, and allow to cook for one more minute.
7. Stir chicken broth, fresh oregano, and the fresh thyme into the pan and stir to combine.
8. Bring the mixture to a boil.
9. Drop the heat to low and allow to simmer for about ten minutes before adding cauliflower and meatballs to it.
10. Allow to cook for about five minutes or until the meatballs are cooked all the way through.
11. Add the spinach to the soup and stir in for about one to two minutes, or until it's sufficiently wilted.
12. Add seasoning as is needed.
13. Serve hot!

Nutrition:
Calories: 420
Carbohydrates: 4 grams
Fat: 26 grams
Protein: 6.5 grams
Soup Recipes

VINAIGRETTE

Preparation Time: 10 minutes
Cooking Time: 10 minutes
Servings: 2
Ingredients:

- · A teaspoon of yellow mustard
- · A spoon of white wine vinegar
- · 1 Teaspoon of honey
- · 165 ml of prepared olive oil:

Directions

1. Mix mustard, vinegar and honey in a bowl.
2. Add a small amount of olive oil and stir until the vinegar thickens.
3. Season with salt and pepper.

Nutrition:
Calories: 1495,
Sodium: 33 mg,
Dietary Fibre: 1.4 g,
Total Fat: 4.3 g,
Total Carbs: 16.2 g,
Protein: 1.5 g.

MEXICAN PORK STEW

Preparation Time: 15 minutes
Cooking Time: 2 hours 10 minutes
Servings: 1
Ingredients:

- 3 tbsp. unsalted butter
- 2½ lb. boneless pork ribs, cut into ¾-inch cubes
- 1 large yellow onion, chopped
- 4 garlic cloves, crushed
- 1½ C. homemade chicken broth
- 2 (10-oz.) cans sugar-free diced tomatoes
- 1 C. canned roasted poblano chiles
- 2 tsp. dried oregano
- 1 tsp. ground cumin
- Salt, to taste
- ¼ C. fresh cilantro, chopped
- 2 tbsp. fresh lime juice

Direction:

1. In a large pan, melt the butter over medium-high heat and cook the pork, onions and garlic for about 5 minutes or until browned.
2. Add the broth and scrape up the browned bits.
3. Add the tomatoes, poblano chiles, oregano, cumin, and salt and bring to a boil.
4. Reduce the heat to medium-low and simmer, covered for about 2 hours.
5. Stir in the fresh cilantro and lime juice and remove from heat.
6. Serve hot.

Nutrition:

Calories: 288

Carbohydrates: 8.8g

Protein: 39.6g

Fat: 10.1g

Sugar: 4g

Sodium: 283mg

Fiber: 2.8g

CURRY SOUP

Preparation Time: 25 minutes
Cooking Time: 20 minutes
Servings: 4
Ingredients:

- ¾ tsp. cumin
- ¼ c. pumpkin seeds, raw
- ½ tsp. garlic powder
- ½ tsp. paprika ½ tsp. sea salt
- 1 c. coconut milk, unsweetened
- 1 clove garlic, minced
- 1 med. onion, diced
- 2 c. carrots, chopped
- 2 tbsp. curry powder
- 3 c. cauliflower, riced
- 3 tbsp. extra virgin olive oil, divided
- 4 c. kale, chopped
- 4 c. vegetable broth
- Sea salt & pepper to taste

Direction:

1. Hear a large saute pan over medium heat with 2 tablespoons of olive oil. Once the oil is hot, add the rice cauliflower to the pan along with the curry powder, cumin, salt, paprika, and garlic powder. Stir thoroughly to combine.
2. While cooking, stir occasionally. Once the cauliflower is warmed through, remove it from the heat.

3. In a large pot over medium heat, add the remainder of your olive oil. Once it's hot, add the onion and allow it to cook for about four minutes. Add the garlic, then cook for about another two minutes.

4. To the large pot, add the broth, kale, carrots, and cauliflower. Stir to thoroughly incorporate.

5. Allow the mixture to come to a boil, drop the heat to low, and allow the soup to simmer for about 15 minutes.

6. Stir the coconut milk into the mixture along with salt and pepper to taste.

7. Garnish with pumpkin seeds and serve hot!

Nutrition:
Calories: 274
Carbs: 11 grams
Fat: 19 grams
Protein: 15 grams

WINTER COMFORT STEW

Preparation Time: 15 minutes
Cooking Time: 50 minutes
Servings: 6
Ingredients:

- 2 tbsp. olive oil
- 1 small yellow onion, chopped
- 2 garlic cloves, chopped
- 2 lb. grass-fed beef chuck, cut into 1-inch cubes
- 1 (14-oz.) can sugar-free crushed tomatoes
- 2 tsp. ground allspice
- 1½ tsp. red pepper flakes
- ½ C. homemade beef broth
- 6 oz. green olives, pitted
- 8 oz. fresh baby spinach
- 2 tbsp. fresh lemon juice
- Salt and freshly ground black pepper, to taste
- ¼ C. fresh cilantro, chopped

Direction:

1. In a pan, heat the oil in a pan over high heat and sauté the onion and garlic for about 2-3 minutes.
2. Add the beef and cook for about 3-4 minutes or until browned, stirring frequently.
3. Add the tomatoes, spices and broth and bring to a boil.
4. Reduce the heat to low and simmer, covered for about 30-40 minutes or until desired doneness of the beef.
5. Stir in the olives and spinach and simmer for about 2-3 minutes.

6. Stir in the lemon juice, salt and black pepper and remove from the heat.

7. Serve hot with the garnishing of cilantro.

Nutrition:

Calories: 388

Carbohydrates: 8g

Protein: 485g

Fat: 17.7g

Sugar: 2.6g

Sodium: 473mg

Fiber: 3.1g

CHAPTER

62

HUNGARIAN PORK STEW

Preparation Time: 15 minutes
Cooking Time: 2 hours 20 minutes
Servings: 10
Ingredients:

- 3 tbsp. olive oil
- 3½ lb. pork shoulder, cut into 4 portions
- 1 tbsp. butter
- 2 medium onions, chopped
- 16 oz. tomatoes, crushed
- 5 garlic cloves, crushed
- 2 Hungarian wax peppers, chopped
- 3 tbsp. Hungarian Sweet paprika
- 1 tbsp. smoked paprika
- 1 tsp. hot paprika
- ½ tsp. caraway seeds
- 1 bay leaf
- 1 C. homemade chicken broth
- 1 packet unflavored gelatin
- 2 tbsp. fresh lemon juice
- Pinch of xanthan gum
- Salt and freshly ground black pepper, to taste

Directions:

1. In a heavy-bottomed pan, heat 1 tbsp. of oil over high heat and sear the pork for about 2-3 minutes or until browned.
2. Transfer the pork onto a plate and cut into bite-sized pieces.

3. In the same pan, heat 1 tbsp. of oil and butter over medium-low heat and sauté the onions for about 5-6 minutes.
4. With a slotted spoon transfer the onion into a bowl.
5. In the same pan, add the tomatoes and cook for about 3-4 minutes, without stirring.
6. Meanwhile, in a small frying pan, heat the remaining oil over-low heat and sauté the garlic, wax peppers, all kinds of paprika and caraway seeds for about 20-30 seconds.
7. Remove from the heat and set aside.
8. In a small bowl, mix together the gelatin and broth.
9. In the large pan, add the cooked pork, garlic mixture, gelatin mixture and bay leaf and bring t0 a gentle boil.
10. Reduce the heat to low and simmer, covered for about 2 hours.
11. Stir in the xanthan gum and simmer for about 3-5 minutes.
12. Stir in the lemon juice, salt and black pepper and remove from the heat.
13. Serve hot.

Nutrition:
Calories: 529
Carbohydrates: 5.8g
Protein: 38.9g
Fat: 38.5g
Sugar: 2.6g
Sodium: 216mg
Fiber: 2.1g

WEEKEND DINNER STEW

Preparation Time: 15 minutes
Cooking Time: 55 minutes
Servings: 6
Ingredients:

- 1½ lb. grass-fed beef stew meat, trimmed and cubed into 1-inch size
- Salt and freshly ground black pepper, to taste
- 1 tbsp. olive oil
- 1 C. homemade tomato puree
- 4 C. homemade beef broth
- 2 C. zucchini, chopped
- 2 celery ribs, sliced
- ½ C. carrots, peeled and sliced
- 2 garlic cloves, minced
- ½ tbsp. dried thyme
- 1 tsp. dried parsley
- 1 tsp. dried rosemary
- 1 tbsp. paprika
- 1 tsp. onion powder
- 1 tsp. garlic powder

Direction:

1. In a large bowl, add the beef cubes, salt and black pepper and toss to coat well.
2. In a large pan, heat the oil over medium-high heat and cook the beef cubes for about 4-5 minutes or until browned.
3. Add the remaining ingredients and stir to combine.
4. Increase the heat to high and bring to a boil.

5. Reduce the heat to low and simmer, covered for about 40-50 minutes.

6. Stir in the salt and black pepper and remove from the heat.

7. Serve hot.

Nutrition:

Calories: 293

Carbohydrates: 8g

Protein: 9.3g

Fat: 10.7g

Sugar: 4g

Sodium: 223mg

Fiber: 2.3g

YELLOW CHICKEN SOUP

Preparation Time: 15 minutes
Cooking Time: 25 minutes
Servings: 5
Ingredients:

- 2½ tsp. ground turmeric
- 1½ tsp. ground cumin
- 1/8 tsp cayenne pepper
- 2 tbsp. butter, divided
- 1 small yellow onion, chopped
- 2 C. cauliflower, chopped
- 2 C. broccoli, chopped
- 4 C. homemade chicken broth
- 1½ C. water
- 1 tsp. fresh ginger root, grated
- 1 bay leaf
- 2 C. Swiss chard, stemmed and chopped finely
- ½ C. unsweetened coconut milk
- 3 (4-oz.) grass-fed boneless, skinless chicken thighs, cut into bite-size pieces
- 2 tbsp. fresh lime juice

Direction:

1. In a small bowl, mix together the turmeric, cumin and cayenne pepper and set aside.
2. Ina large pan, melt 1 tbsp. of the butter over medium heat and sauté the onion for about 3-4 minutes.
3. Add the cauliflower, broccoli and half of the spice mixture and cook for another 3-4 minutes.

4. Add the broth, water, ginger and bay leaf and bring to a boil.
5. Reduce the heat to low and simmer for about 8-10 minutes.
6. Stir in the Swiss chard and coconut milk and cook for about 1-2 minutes.
7. Meanwhile, in a large skillet, melt the remaining butter over medium heat and sear the chicken pieces for about 5 minutes.
8. Stir in the remaining spice mix and cook for about 5 minutes, stirring frequently.
9. Transfer the soup into serving bowls and top with the chicken pieces.
10. Drizzle with lime juice and serve.

Nutrition:
Calories: 258
Carbohydrates: 8.4g
Protein: 18.4g
Fat: 16.8g
Sugar: 3g
Sodium: 753mg
Fiber: 2.9g

IDEAL COLD WEATHER STEW

Preparation Time: 20 minutes
Cooking Time: 2 hours 40 minutes
Servings: 6
Ingredients:

- 3 tbsp. olive oil, divided
- 8 oz. fresh mushrooms, quartered
- 1¼ lb. grass-fed beef chuck roast, trimmed and cubed into 1-inch size
- 2 tbsp. tomato paste
- ½ tsp. dried thyme
- 1 bay leaf
- 5 C. homemade beef broth
- 6 oz. celery root, peeled and cubed
- 4 oz. yellow onions, chopped roughly
- 3 oz. carrot, peeled and sliced
- 2 garlic cloves, sliced
- Salt and freshly ground black pepper, to taste

Direction:

1. In a Dutch oven, heat 1 tbsp. of the oil over medium heat and cook the mushrooms for about 2 minutes, without stirring.
2. Stir the mushroom and cook for about 2 minutes more.
3. With a slotted spoon, transfer the mushroom onto a plate.
4. In the same pan, heat the remaining oil over medium-high heat and sear the beef cubes for about 4-5 minutes.
5. Stir in the tomato paste, thyme and bay leaf and cook for about 1 minute.
6. Stir in the broth and bring to a boil.

7. Reduce the heat to low and simmer, covered for about 1½ hours.
8. Stir in the mushrooms, celery, onion, carrot and garlic and simmers for about 40-60 minutes.
9. Stir in the salt and black pepper and remove from the heat.
10. Serve hot.

Nutrition:
Calories: 447
Carbohydrates: 7.4g
Protein: 30.8g
Fat: 32.3g
Sugar: 8g
Sodium: 764mg
Fiber: 1.9g

DELICIOUS TOMATO BASIL SOUP

Preparation Time: 10 minutes
Cooking Time: 40 minutes
Servings: 4
Ingredients:

- ¼ c. olive oil
- ½ c. heavy cream
- 1 lb. tomatoes, fresh
- 4 c. chicken broth, divided
- 4 cloves garlic, fresh
- Sea salt & pepper to taste

Direction:

1. Preheat oven to 400° Fahrenheit and line a baking sheet with foil.
2. Remove the cores from your tomatoes and place them on the baking sheet along with the cloves of garlic.
3. Drizzle tomatoes and garlic with olive oil, salt, and pepper.
4. Roast at 400° Fahrenheit for 30 minutes.
5. Pull the tomatoes out of the oven and place into a blender, along with the juices that have dripped onto the pan during roasting.
6. Add two cups of the chicken broth to the blender.
7. Blend until smooth, then strain the mixture into a large saucepan or a pot.
8. While the pan is on the stove, whisk the remaining two cups of broth and the cream into the soup.
9. Simmer for about ten minutes.
10. Season to taste, then serve hot!

Nutrition:
Calories: 225
Carbohydrates: 5.5 grams
Fat: 20 grams
Protein: 6.5 grams

Tomato and broccoli soup

Preparation Time: 50 minutes
Cooking Time: 55 minutes
Servings: 4
Ingredients:

- A drizzle of olive oil
- Canned sugar-free tomatoes- 28 oz.
- Crushed red pepper- ¼ tsp.
- Broccoli head: into florets- 1
- Small ginger: chopped- 1
- Onion: chopped – 1
- Garlic clove: minced- 1
- Coriander seeds- 2 tsp.
- Black pepper
- Salt

Directions:

1. Boil water and salt in a pan on medium-high and add broccoli florets to steam for 2 minutes.
2. Remove and put in a bowl of ice water. Drain and set aside.
3. Heat pan and put in coriander seeds to toast for 4 minutes. Blend in a blender and set aside.
4. Pour olive oil in a pot and set to medium and add red pepper, salt, pepper and onions and cook for 7 minutes.
5. Mix in coriander seeds and garlic and let it cook for 3 minutes.
6. Pour in tomatoes and let simmer for 10 minutes.
7. Mix in broccoli and cook for 12 minutes.
8. Serve

Nutrition:
Calories- 152, carbs- 1, protein- 9, fiber- 8, fats- 9

BOK CHOY STIR FRY WITH FRIED BACON SLICES

Preparation Time: 17 minutes

Cooking Time: 15 minutes

Servings: 2

Ingredients:

- Bok choy; chopped - 2 cup.
- Garlic cloves; minced - 2
- Bacon slices; chopped - 2
- A drizzle of avocado oil
- Salt and black pepper to the taste.

Instructions:

1. Take a pan and heat it with oil over medium heat.
2. When the oil is hot, add bacon and keep stirring it until it's brown and crispy.
3. Transfer them to paper towels to drain out the excess oil.
4. Now bring the pan to medium heat and in it add garlic and bok choy.
5. Again give it a stir and cook it for 5 minutes.
6. Now drizzle and add some salt, pepper and the fried bacon and stir them for another 1 minute.
7. Turn off the heat and divide them in plates to serve.

Nutrition
Calories: 50; Fat: 1; Fiber: 1; Carbs: 2; Protein: 2

BROCCOLI-CAULIFLOWER STEW

Preparation Time: 25 minutes

Cooking Time: 15 minutes

Servings: 5

Ingredients:

· Bacon slices: chopped -2
· Cauliflower head: separated into florets- 1
· Broccoli head: separated into florets- 1
· Butter- 2 tbsp.
· Garlic cloves: minced- 2
· Salt
· Black pepper

Directions:

1. Put a pan on medium heat and dissolve the butter and the garlic. Add the bacon slices to brown for 3 minutes all over.
2. Mix in broccoli and cauliflower florets to cook for 2 minutes.
3. Pour water over it and cover the lid and let cook for 10 minutes.
4. Season with pepper and salt and puree soup with a dipping blend.
5. Let boil slowly for some minutes on medium heat.
6. Serve into bowls.

Nutrition:

Calories- 128, carbs- 4, protein- 6, fiber- 7, fats- 2

CREAMY AVOCADO SOUP

Preparation Time: 20 minutes
Cooking Time: 15 minutes
Servings: 4
Ingredients:

- Chicken stock, 3 c.
- Black pepper
- Chopped scallions, 2
- Salt
- Heavy cream, 2/3 c.
- Butter, 2 tbsps.
- Chopped avocados, 2

Directions:

1. Over a medium source of heat, set the saucepan and cook the scallions for 2 minutes
2. Stir in 2 ½ cups stock to simmer for 3 minutes
3. Set the blender in position to blend avocados, heavy cream, the remaining stock, and seasonings.
4. Return to a pan to cook for 2 minutes as you adjust the seasoning
5. Serve in soup bowls

Nutrition:
Calories: 335, Fat: 32, Fiber: 9, Carbs: 13, Protein: 3

BOK CHOY MUSHROOM SOUP

Preparation Time: 25 minutes

Cooking Time: 15 minutes

Servings: 4

Ingredients:

· Bacon strips: chopped- 2
· Beef stock- 3 cups
· Bok choy: chopped- 1 bunch
· Onion: chopped- 1
· Parmesan cheese: grated- 3 tbsp.
· Coconut aminos- 3 tbsp.
· Worcestershire sauce- 2 tbsp.
· Red pepper flakes- ½ tbsp.
· Mushrooms: chopped- 1½ cups
· Black Pepper
· Salt

Directions:

1. Put bacon in a saucepan over medium-high heat to brown until crispy then remove to paper towels to drain.
2. To medium heat, add the mushrooms and onions in the pan and cook for 15 minutes.
3. Pour in the stock, pepper flakes, aminos, bok choy, Worcestershire sauce, salt and pepper and mix.
4. Cook until bok choy is tender.
5. Serve into bowls and sprinkle with Parmesan cheese and bacon.

Nutrition:

Calories- 100, carbs- 1, protein- 5, fiber- 9, fats- 5

TASTY RADISH SOUP

Preparation Time: 30 minutes

Cooking Time: 45 minutes

Servings: 4

Ingredients:

· Chopped onion, 1
· Salt
· Chopped celery stalk, 2
· Chicken stock, 6 c.
· Coconut oil, 3 tbsps.
· Quartered radishes, 2 bunches
· Black pepper
· Minced garlic cloves, 6

Directions:

1. Set the pan over medium heat and melt the oil
2. Stir in the celery, onion, and garlic to cook until soft, about 5 minutes
3. Stir in the stock, radishes, and seasonings.
4. Cover and simmer to boil for 15 minutes
5. Enjoy while still hot

Nutrition:

Calories: 131, Fat: 12, Fiber: 8, Carbs: 4, Protein: 1

FRIED GARLICY BACON AND BOK CHOY BROTH

Preparation Time: 17 minutes
Cooking Time: 15 minutes
Servings: 2
Ingredients:

- Bok choy: chopped- 2 cups
- A drizzle of avocado oil
- Bacon slices: chopped- 2
- Garlic cloves: minced- 2
- Black pepper
- Salt

Directions:

1. Put bacon in a pan on medium heat and let crisp. Remove and let drain on paper towels.
2. Add bok choy and garlic to the pan and let cook for 4 minutes.
3. Season with pepper and salt and put the bacon back into the pan.
4. Let cook for 1 minute and serve.

Nutrition:
Calories- 116, carbs- 8, protein- 3, fiber- 8, fats- 1

NUTRITIONAL MUSTARD GREENS AND SPINACH SOUP

Preparation Time: 25 minutes

Cooking Time: 15 minutes

Servings: 6

Ingredients:

· Spinach; torn - 5 cups.
· Fenugreek seeds - 1/2 teaspoon.
· Cumin seeds - 1 teaspoon.
· Jalapeno; chopped - 1 tablespoon.
· Mustard greens; chopped - 5 cups.
· Ghee - 2 teaspoons.
· Paprika - 1/2 teaspoon.
· Avocado oil - 1 tablespoon.
· Coriander seeds - 1 teaspoon.
· Yellow onion; chopped - 1 cup.
· Garlic; minced - 1 tablespoon.
· Ginger; grated - 1 tablespoon.
· Turmeric; ground - 1/2 teaspoon.
· Coconut milk - 3 cups.
· Salt and black pepper to the taste.

Directions:

1. Add coriander, fenugreek and cumin seed in a heated pot with oil over medium high heat.
2. Now stir and brow them for 2 minutes.
3. In the same pot, add onions and again stir them for 3 minutes.

4. Now after the onion's cooked, add half of the garlic, jalapenos, ginger and turmeric.
5. Again, give it a good stir and cook for another 3 minutes.
6. Add some more mustard greens, spinach and saute everything for 10 minutes.
7. After it's done add milk, salt, pepper before blending the soup with an immersion blender.
8. Now take another pan and heat it up over medium heat with some ghee drizzled on it.
9. In it, add garlic, paprika, and give it a good stir before turning off the heat.
10. Bring the soup to heat over medium heat and transfer them into soup bowls.
11. Top it with some drizzles of ghee and paprika. Now it's ready to serve hot.

Nutrition:
Calories: - 143; Fat: 6; Fiber: 3; Carbs: 7; Protein: 7

HASH BROWNS WITH RADISH

Preparation Time: 20 minutes
Cooking Time: 15 minutes
Servings: 4
Ingredients:

· Shredded Parmesan cheese, 1/3 c.
· Garlic powder, ½ tsp.
· Salt
· Shredded radishes, 1 lb.
· Black pepper
· Onion powder, ½ tsp.
· Medium eggs, 4

Directions:

1. Set a large mixing bowl in a working surface.
2. Combine the seasonings, radishes, eggs, onion, and parmesan cheese
3. Arrange the mixture in a well-lined baking tray.
4. Set the oven for 10 minutes at 3750F. Allow to bake
5. Enjoy while still hot

Nutrition:
Calories: 104, Fat: 6, Fiber: 8, Carbs: 5, Protein: 6

BAKED RADISHES

Preparation Time: 30 minutes

Cooking Time: 35 minutes

Servings: 4

Ingredients:

· Chopped chives, 1 tbsp.
· Sliced radishes, 15
· Salt
· Vegetable oil cooking spray
· Black pepper

Directions:

1. Line your baking sheet well then spray with the cooking spray
2. Set the sliced radishes on the baking tray then sprinkle with cooking oil
3. Add the seasonings then top with chives
4. Set the oven for 10 minutes at 375oF, allow to bake
5. Turn the radishes to bake for 10 minutes
6. Serve cold

Nutrition:
Calories: 63, Fat: 8, Fiber: 3, Carbs: 6, Protein: 1

COLESLAW AVOCADO SALAD

Preparation Time: 10 minutes

Cooking Time: 15 minutes

Servings: 4

Ingredients:

· White vinegar, 1 tbsp.

· Salt

· Olive oil, 2 tbsps.

· Black pepper

· Lemon stevia, ¼ tsp.

· Juice from 2 limes

· Mashed avocados, 2

· Chopped onion, ¼ c.

· Chopped cilantro, ¼ c.

· For coleslaw mix

· Salt, 1 tsp.

· Small red cabbage, ¼

· Shredded carrot, ½

· Lemon juice, ¼ c.

· Small green cabbage, ½

· Olive oil, ¼ c.

· Stevia, 1 tbsp.

· Zest of ½ lemon

Directions:

1. Set the mixing bowl in place to make the coleslaw salad

2. Add the mashed avocado and onions to coat well

3. Combine the seasonings, lime juice, vinegar, stevia, and oil in another bowl.

4. Add the mixture to the salad, mix to coat evenly

5. Enjoy

Nutrition:

Calories: 481, Fat: 42, Fiber: 12, Carbs: 26, Protein: 6

SHERRY WATERCRESS BROTH

Preparation Time: 20 minutes

Cooking Time: 15 minutes

Servings: 4

Ingredients:

- Sherry - ¼ cup
- Watercress- 6½ cups
- Chicken stock- 6 cups
- Coconut aminos- 2 tsp.
- Whisked egg whites of 3 eggs
- Shallots: chopped- 3
- Sesame seeds- 2 tsp.
- Salt and pepper

Directions:

1. Pour the stock into the pot and add sherry, coconut amino, salt and pepper and mix. Boil on medium heat.
2. Mix in watercress, shallots, and whisked whites and let boil.
3. Serve sprinkled with sesame seeds.

Nutrition:

Calories- 73, carbs- 7, protein- 9, fiber- 2, fats- 7

CREAMED CHEDDAR RADISHES

Preparation Time: 35 minutes

Cooking Time: 15 minutes

Servings: 1

Ingredients:

· Black pepper
· Halved radishes, 7 oz.
· Bacon slices, 2
· Chopped green onion, 1 tbsp.
· Sour cream, 2 tbsps.
· Cayenne pepper powder
· Salt
· Grated cheddar cheese, 1 tbsp.

Directions:

1. Set the radishes in a saucepan then add water.
2. Let it boil for 10 minutes over medium heat then drain the water
3. Set your pan over medium-high heat to cook the bacon to a crispy texture.
4. Drain the excess grease in a paper towel and reserve
5. Set the same pan again over medium heat then stir-fry the radishes for seven minutes
6. Stir in the seasonings, sour cream, and cayenne pepper powder for 7 minutes
7. Serve with crumbled bacon topped with cheddar cheese

Nutrition:

Calories: 319, Fat: 25, Fiber: 3, Carbs: 8, Protein: 11

MUSTARD EGG AND AVOCADO SALAD

Preparation Time: 17 minutes

Cooking Time: 15 minutes

Servings: 4

Ingredients:

· Salt
· Mayonnaise, ¼ c.
· Medium eggs, 4
· Sliced avocado, 1
· Mustard, 2 tsps.
· Mixed lettuce leaves, 4 c.
· Chopped chives, 1 tbsp.
· Black pepper
· Minced garlic cloves, 2

Directions:

1. Set the cooking pan over medium-high heat.
2. Add water, eggs, and salt then allow to boil for about 7minutes.
3. Once boiled, drain the liquid, let cool then chop them.
4. Set a salad bowl in position to mix lettuce eggs and avocado
5. Toss with garlic, seasonings, and chives to coat
6. Combine the seasonings, mustard, and mayonnaise in another bowl
7. Add to the salad, toss and serve.

Nutrition:

Calories: 278, Fat: 16, Fiber: 7, Carbs: 13, Protein: 12

CUCUMBER AVOCADO SALAD MIX

Preparation Time: 10 minutes
Cooking Time: 15 minutes
Servings: 4
Ingredients:

- Salt
- Sliced cucumber, 1
- Chopped avocados, 2
- Olive oil, 2 tbsps.
- Sliced onion, 1
- Chopped cilantro, ¼ c.
- Lemon juice, 2 tbsps.
- Black pepper
- Halved cherry tomatoes, 1 lb.

Directions:

1. Stir together cucumber, tomatoes, avocado, and onion in a salad bowl
2. Add the seasonings, lemon juice, and oil. Mix to coat well.
3. Serve cold topped with cilantro

Nutrition:
Calories: 310, Fat: 27, Fiber: 1, Carbs: 16, Protein: 8

FRIED EGGS WITH KALE AND BACON

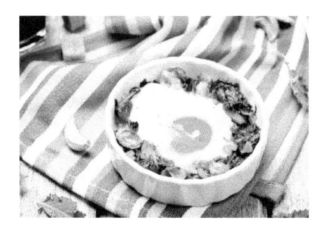

Preparation Time 5 minutes

Cooking Time: 15 minutes

Servings: 2

Ingredients

- · 4 slices of turkey bacon, chopped
- · 1 bunch of kale, chopped
- · 3 oz. butter, unsalted
- · 2 eggs
- · 2 tbsp. chopped walnuts
- · Seasoning:
- · 1/3 tsp salt
- · 1/3 tsp ground black pepper

Directions:

1. Take a frying pan, place it over medium heat, add two-third of the butter in it, and let it melt, then add kale, switch heat to medium-high level and cook for 4 to 5 minutes until edges have turned golden brown.
2. When done, transfer kale to a plate, set aside until required, add bacon into the pan and cook for 4 minutes until crispy.
3. Return kale into the pan, add nuts, stir until mixed and cook for 2 minutes until thoroughly warmed.
4. Transfer kale into the bowl, add remaining butter into the pan, crack eggs into the pan and fry them for 2 to 3 minutes until cooked to the desired level.
5. Distribute kale between two plates, add fried eggs on the side, sprinkle with salt and black pepper, and then serve.

Nutrition: 525 Calories; 50 g Fats; 14.4 g Protein; 1.1 g Net Carb; 2.8 g Fiber;

EGGS WITH GREENS

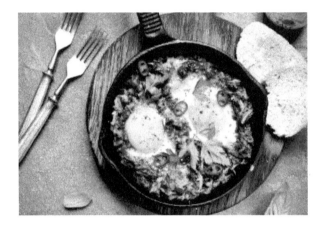

Preparation Time: 5 minutes

Cooking Time: 10 minutes;

Servings: 2

Ingredients

- 3 tbsp. chopped parsley
- 3 tbsp. chopped cilantro
- ¼ tsp cayenne pepper
- 2 eggs
- 1 tbsp. butter, unsalted
- Seasoning:
- ¼ tsp salt
- 1/8 tsp ground black pepper

Directions:

1. Take a medium skillet pan, place it over medium-low heat, add butter and wait until it melts.

2. Then add parsley and cilantro, season with salt and black pepper, stir until mixed and cook for 1 minute.
3. Make two space in the pan, crack an egg into each space, and then sprinkle with cayenne pepper, cover the pan with the lid and cook for 2 to 3 minutes until egg yolks have set.
4. Serve.

Nutrition: 135 Calories; 11.1 g Fats; 7.2 g Protein; 0.2 g Net Carb; 0.5 g Fiber;

SPICY CHAFFLE WITH JALAPENO

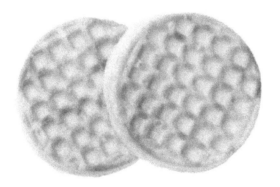

Preparation Time: 5 minutes
Cooking Time: 10 minutes;
Servings: 2
Ingredients

- 2 tsp coconut flour
- ½ tbsp. chopped jalapeno pepper
- 2 tsp cream cheese
- 1 egg
- 2 oz. shredded mozzarella cheese
- Seasoning:
- ¼ tsp salt
- 1/8 tsp ground black pepper

Directions:

1. Switch on a mini waffle maker and let it preheat for 5 minutes.
2. Meanwhile, take a medium bowl, place all the ingredients in it and then mix by using an immersion blender until smooth.

3. Ladle the batter evenly into the waffle maker, shut with lid, and let it cook for 3 to 4 minutes until firm and golden brown.
4. Serve.

Nutrition: 153 Calories; 10.7 g Fats; 11.1 g Protein; 1 g Net Carb; 1 g Fiber;

BULLETPROOF TEA

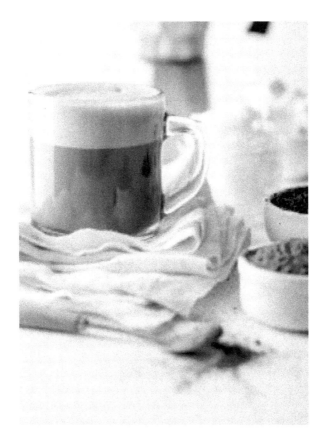

Preparation Time: 5 minutes

Cooking Time: 0 minutes

Servings: 2

Ingredients

- ¼ tsp cinnamon
- 2 cups strong tea
- 2 tbsp. coconut oil

· 2 tbsp. coconut milk

Directions:

1. Distribute tea between two mugs, add remaining ingredients evenly and then stir until blended.
2. Serve.

Nutrition: 151 Calories; 17 g Fats; 0 g Protein; 1 g Net Carb; 0 g Fiber;

TEA WITH COCONUT

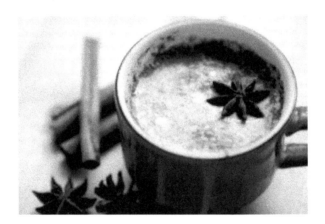

Preparation Time: 10 minutes

Cooking Time: 0 minutes;

Servings 2

Ingredients

- 2 tea bags, cinnamon-flavored
- 2 tbsp. MCT oil
- ¼ cup coconut milk, unsweetened
- 2 cups boiling water

Directions:

1. Pour boiling water between two mugs, add a tea into each mug and let them steep for 5 minutes.
2. Meanwhile, take a small saucepan, place it over medium heat, pour in milk and heat for 3 minutes or more until hot.
3. After 5 minutes, remove tea bags from mugs, stir in milk, and MCT oil by using a milk frother until combined and then serve.

Nutrition: 191 Calories; 16 g Fats; 11 g Protein; 2 g Net Carb; 0 g Fiber;

CAULIFLOWER AND EGG PLATE

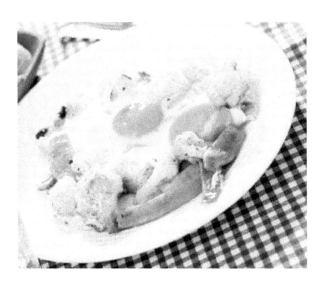

Preparation Time: 5 minutes

Cooking Time: 12 minutes;

Servings: 2

Ingredients

- · 4 oz. cauliflower florets, chopped
- · 1 jalapeno pepper, sliced
- · 2 eggs
- · 1 ½ tbsp. avocado oil
- · Seasoning:
- · ¼ tsp salt
- · 1/8 tsp ground black pepper

Directions:

1. Take a skillet pan, place it over medium heat, add oil and when hot, add cauliflower florets and jalapeno and then cook for 5 to 7 minutes until tender.
2. Make two spaces in the pan, crack an egg in each space, and then cook for 3 to 4 minutes until eggs have cooked to the desired level.
3. When done, sprinkle salt and black pepper over eggs and then serve.

Nutrition: 191 Calories; 16 g Fats; 11 g Protein; 2 g Net Carb; 0 g Fiber

BUTTERNUT SQUASH AND GREEN ONIONS WITH EGGS

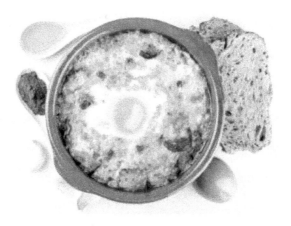

Preparation Time: 5 minutes
Cooking Time: 8 minutes;
Servings: 2
Ingredients

- · 4 oz. butternut squash pieces
- · 1 green onion, sliced
- · ½ tbsp. butter, unsalted
- · 2 tsp grated parmesan cheese
- · 2 eggs
- · Seasoning:
- · ¼ tsp salt
- · ¼ tsp ground black pepper
- · 1 tsp avocado oil

Directions:

1. Take a skillet pan, place it over medium heat, add butter and oil and when hot, add butternut squash and green onion, season with 1/8 tsp of each salt and black pepper, stir until mixed and cook for 3 to 5 minutes until tender.
2. Make two space in the pan, crack an egg in each space, and sprinkle with cheese, season with remaining salt and black pepper, cover with the lid and cook for 2 to 3 minutes until the egg has cooked to the desired level.
3. Serve.

Nutrition: 191 Calories; 16 g Fats; 11 g Protein; 2 g Net Carb; 0 g Fiber

BROCCOLI, ASPARAGUS AND CHEESE FRITTATA

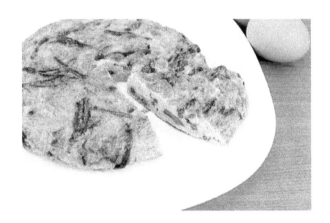

Preparation Time: 5 minutes

Cooking Time: 16 minutes;

Servings: 2

Ingredients

- ¼ cup chopped broccoli florets
- 1-ounce asparagus spear cuts
- ½ tsp garlic powder
- 2 tbsp. whipping cream
- 2 eggs
- Seasoning:
- 2 tsp tbsp. avocado oil
- 1/8 tsp salt
- 1/8 tsp ground black pepper

Directions:

1. Turn on the oven, then set it to 350 degrees F and let it preheat.
2. Take a medium bowl, crack eggs in it, add salt, black pepper and cream, whisk until combined and then stir in cheese, set aside until required.
3. Take a medium skillet pan, place it over medium heat, add oil and when hot, add broccoli florets and asparagus, sprinkle with garlic powder, stir until mixed and cook for 3 to 4 minutes until tender.
4. Spread the vegetables evenly in the pan, pour egg mixture over them and cook for 1 to 2 minutes until the mixture begins to firm.
5. Transfer the pan into the oven and then cook for 10 to 12 minutes until frittata has cooked and the top has turned golden brown.
6. When done, cut the frittata into slices and then serve.

Nutrition: 206 Calories; 17 g Fats; 10 g Protein; 2 g Net Carb; 1 g Fiber;

BROCCOLI AND EGG PLATE

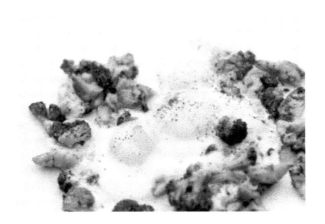

Preparation Time: 5 minutes

Cooking Time: 5 minutes;

Servings: 2

Ingredients

- 3 oz. broccoli florets, chopped
- 2 eggs
- 1 tbsp. avocado oil
- ¼ tsp salt
- 1/8 tsp ground black pepper

Directions:

1. Take a heatproof bowl, place broccoli florets in it, cover with a plastic wrap, microwave for 2 minutes, and then drain well.
2. Take a medium skillet pan, place it over medium heat, add oil and when hot, add broccoli florets and cook for 2 minutes until golden brown.

3. Spread broccoli florets evenly in the pan crack eggs in the pan, sprinkle with salt and black pepper, cover with the lid and cook for 2 to 3 minutes until eggs have cooked to the desired level.

4. Serve.

Nutrition: 155 Calories; 12 g Fats; 8 g Protein; 1.6 g Net Carb; 1 g Fiber;

CHAPTER

90

RADISH WITH FRIED EGGS

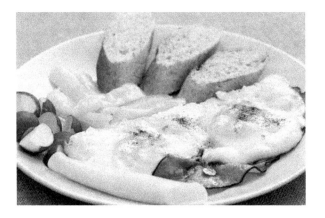

Preparation Time: 5 minutes

Cooking Time: 10 minutes;

Servings: 2

Ingredients

- ½ bunch of radish, diced
- ½ tsp garlic powder
- 1 tbsp. butter
- 1 tbsp. avocado oil
- 2 eggs
- Seasoning:
- 1/3 tsp salt
- ¼ tsp ground black pepper

Directions:

1. Take a medium skillet pan, place it over medium heat, add butter and when it melts, add radish, sprinkle with garlic powder and ¼ tsp salt and cook for 5 minutes until tender.
2. Distribute radish between two plates, then return pan over medium heat, add oil and when hot, crack eggs in it and fry for 2 to 3 minutes until cooked to desired level.
3. Add eggs to the radish and then serve.

Nutrition: 187 Calories; 17 g Fats; 7 g Protein; 0.4 g Net Carb; 0.5 g Fiber;

SUNNY SIDE UP EGGS ON CREAMED SPINACH

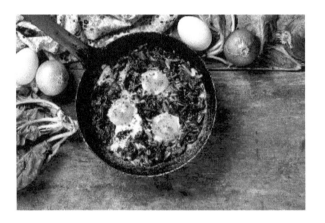

Preparation Time: 5 minutes

Cooking Time: 10 minutes;

Servings: 2

Ingredients

- 4 oz. of spinach leaves
- 1 tbsp. mustard paste
- 4 tbsp. whipping cream
- 2 eggs
- Seasoning:
- ¼ tsp salt
- ¼ tsp ground black pepper
- ½ tsp dried thyme
- 1 tbsp. avocado oil

Directions:

1. Take a medium skillet pan, place it over high heat, pour in water to cover its bottom, then add spinach, toss until mixed and cook for 2 minutes until spinach wilts.
2. Then drain the spinach by passing it through a sieve placed on a bowl and set it aside.
3. Take a medium saucepan, place it over medium heat, add spinach, mustard, thyme, and cream, stir until mixed and cook for 2 minutes.
4. Then sprinkle black pepper over spinach, stir until mixed and remove the pan from heat.
5. Take a medium skillet pan, place it over medium-high heat, add oil and when hot, crack eggs in it and fry for 3 to 4 minutes until eggs have cooked to the desired level.
6. Divide spinach mixture evenly between two plates, top with a fried egg and then serve.

Nutrition: 280 Calories; 23.3 g Fats; 10.2 g Protein; 2.7 g Net Carb; 2.8 g Fiber;

CREAMY KALE BAKED EGGS

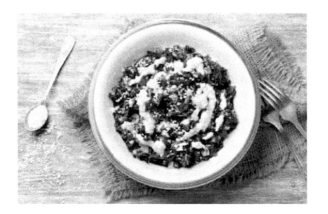

Preparation Time: 10 minutes

Cooking Time: 20 minutes

Servings: 2

Ingredients

- · 1 bunch of kale, chopped
- · 1-ounce grape tomatoes, halved
- · 3 tbsp. whipping cream
- · 2 tbsp. sour cream
- · 2 eggs
- · Seasoning:
- · ½ tsp salt
- · ½ tsp ground black pepper
- · ½ tsp Italian seasoning
- · 1 ½ tbsp. butter, unsalted

Directions:

1. Turn on the oven, then set it to 400 degrees F and let it preheat.
2. Meanwhile, take a medium skillet pan, place butter in it, add butter and when it melts, add kale and cook for 2 minutes until wilted
3. Add Italian seasoning, 1/3 tsp each of salt and black pepper, cream and sour cream, then stir until mixed and cook for2 minutes until cheese has melted and the kale has thickened slightly.
4. Take two ramekins, divide creamed kale evenly between them, then top with cherry tomatoes and carefully crack an egg into each ramekin.
5. Sprinkle remaining salt and black pepper on eggs and then bake for 15 minutes until eggs have cooked completely.
6. Serve.

Nutrition: 301.5 Calories; 25.5 g Fats; 9.8 g Protein; 4.3 g Net Carb; 4 g Fiber;

BUTTER ASPARAGUS WITH CREAMY EGGS

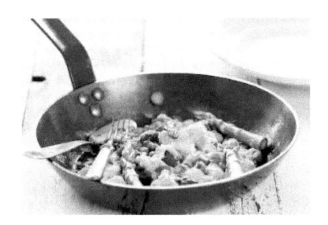

Preparation Time: 5 minutes

Cooking Time: 8 minutes;

Servings: 2

Ingredients

- · 4 oz. asparagus
- · 2 eggs, blended
  1. oz. grated parmesan cheese
- · 1-ounce sour cream
- · 2 tbsp. butter, unsalted
- · Seasoning:
- · 1/3 tsp salt
- · 1/8 tsp ground black pepper
- · ¼ tsp cayenne pepper
- · ½ tbsp. avocado oil

Directions:

1. Take a medium skillet pan, place it over medium heat, add butter and when it melts, add blended eggs and then cook for 2 to 3 minutes until scrambled to the desired level; don't overcook.
2. Spoon the scrambled eggs into a food processor, add 1/8 tsp salt, cayenne pepper, sour cream and cheese and then pulse for 1 minute until smooth.
3. Return skillet pan over medium heat, add oil and when hot, add asparagus, season with black pepper and remaining salt, toss until mixed and cook for 3 minutes or more until roasted.
4. Distribute asparagus between two plates, add egg mixture, and then serve.

Nutrition: 338 Calories; 28.5 g Fats; 14.4 g Protein; 4.7 g Net Carb; 1.2 g Fiber;

SPINACH EGG MUFFINS

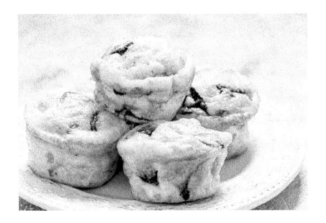

Preparation Time: 5 minutes

Cooking Time: 10 minutes;

Servings: 2

Ingredients

- ½ cups chopped spinach
- 1/8 tsp dried basil
- 1/8 tsp garlic powder
- 2 large eggs
- 3 tbsp. grated Parmesan cheese
- Seasoning:
- ¼ tsp of sea salt
- 1/8 tsp ground black pepper

Directions:

1. Turn on the oven, then set it to 400 degrees F, and let preheat.

2. Meanwhile, place eggs in a bowl, season with salt and black pepper and whisk until blended.

3. Add garlic and basil, whisk in mixed and then stir in spinach and cheese until combined.

4. Take two silicone muffin cups, grease them with reserved bacon greased, fill them evenly with prepared egg mixture and bake for 8 to 10 minutes until the top has nicely browned.

5. Serve.

Nutrition: 55 Calories; 3.5 g Fats; 4.5 g Protein; 0.4 g Net Carb; 0.2 g Fiber;

BROCCOLI AND EGG MUFFIN

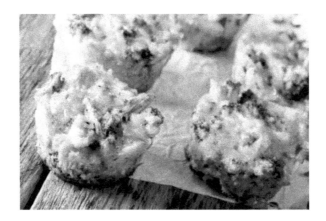

Preparation Time: 10 minutes;
Cooking Time: 10 minutes
Servings: 2
Ingredients

- ¼ cup broccoli florets, steamed, chopped
- 2 tbsp. grated cheddar cheese
- 1/16 tsp dried thyme
- 1/16 tsp garlic powder
- 1 egg
- Seasoning:
- ¼ tsp salt
- 1/8 tsp ground black pepper

Directions:

1. Turn on the oven, then set it to 400 degrees F and let it preheat.

2. Meanwhile, take two silicone muffin cups, grease them with oil, and evenly fill them with broccoli and cheese.
3. Crack the egg in a bowl, add garlic powder, thyme, salt, and black pepper, whisk well, then evenly pour the mixture into muffin cups and bake for 8 to 10 minutes until done.
4. Serve.

Nutrition: 76 Calories; 5.1 g Fats; 5.7 g Protein; 1.2 g Net Carb; 0.7 g Fiber;

JALAPENO AND CHEESE EGG MUFFINS

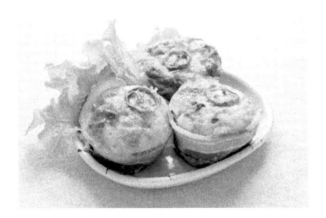

Preparation Time: 10 minutes
Cooking Time: 15 minutes
Servings: 2
Ingredients

- · 1 jalapeno pepper, diced
- · 2 tbsp. sliced green onions
- · 2 tbsp. grated parmesan cheese
- · 1 tsp all-purpose seasoning
- · 2 eggs
- · Seasoning:
- · 1/3 tsp salt
- · ¼ tsp ground black pepper

Directions:

1. Turn on the oven, then set it to 375 degrees F, and let it preheat.

2. Meanwhile, take two silicone muffin cups, grease with oil, and evenly fill them with cheese, jalapeno pepper, and green onion.

3. Crack eggs in a bowl, season with salt, black pepper, and all-purpose seasoning, whisk well, then evenly pour the mixture into muffin cups and bake for 15 to 20 minutes or until the top is slightly brown and muffins have puffed up.

4. Serve.

Nutrition: 108 Calories; 7.1 g Fats; 8.9 g Protein; 1.8 g Net Carb; 0.4 g Fiber;

CHEESY TOMATO AND OLIVE MUFFINS

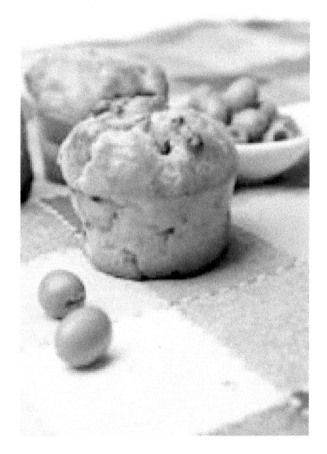

Preparation Time: 10 minutes
Cooking Time: 12 minutes;
Servings: 2
Ingredients

- 4 1/3 tbsp. almond flour
- ½ tbsp. coconut flour
- 1/3 tbsp. chopped tomato
- 1/3 tbsp. sliced green olives
- 2 tbsp. sour cream
- Seasoning:
- 1/8 tsp baking powder
- 2/3 tbsp. avocado oil
- 3 tbsp. grated parmesan cheese
- ½ of egg

Directions:

1. Turn on the oven, then set it to 320 degrees F and let it preheat.
2. Meanwhile, take a medium bowl, place flours in it, and stir in the baking powder until mixed.
3. Add eggs along with sour cream and oil, whisk until blended and then fold in cheese, tomato, and olives until just mixed.
4. Take two silicone muffin cups, add the prepared batter in it evenly and then bake for 10 to 12 minutes until cooked but slightly moist in the middle.
5. When done, let muffin cools for 5 minutes, then take them out and serve.

Nutrition: 256 Calories; 23.5 g Fats; 8.7 g Protein; 1 g Net Carb; 1.8 g Fiber;

BUTTERY BROCCOLI AND BACON

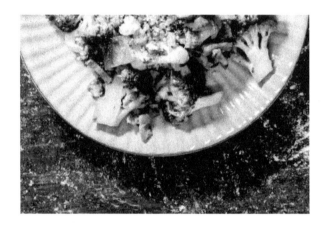

Preparation Time: 5 minutes;

Cooking Time: 12 minutes;

Servings: 2

Ingredients

1 slice of turkey bacon

1 cup chopped broccoli florets

1/8 tsp garlic powder

¼ tsp Italian seasoning

¼ tbsp. unsalted butter

Seasoning:

1/8 tsp salt

1/8 tsp ground black pepper

Directions:

1. Take a medium skillet pan, place it over high heat, add bacon slice and cook for 3 to 5 minutes until crispy.
2. Transfer bacon to a cutting board and then chop it into small pieces.

3. Reduce the heat to medium-low level, add broccoli florets into the pan, stir well into the bacon grease, add butter, then toss until mixed and cook for 5 minutes until tender.
4. Season the broccoli florets with salt, black pepper, and Italian seasoning, add chopped bacon, stir well and cook for 2 minutes until thoroughly heated.
5. Serve.

Nutrition: 77 Calories; 5 g Fats; 5 g Protein; 1 g Net Carb; 2 g Fiber;

BROCCOLI SALAD WITH BACON

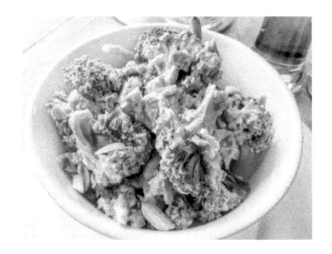

Preparation Time: 5 minutes;

Cooking Time: 0 minutes;

Servings: 2

Ingredients

- · 1 cup broccoli florets, chopped
- · 4 tbsp. whipped topping
- · 2 tbsp. shredded cheddar cheese
- · 3 slices of turkey bacon, cooked, chopped
- · 1/3 tsp garlic powder
- · Seasoning:
- · 1/8 tsp salt
- · 1/8 tsp dried parsley

Directions:

1. Take a medium bowl, place whipped topping in it, whisk in garlic powder and parsley, and then fold in broccoli florets.
2. Top with bacon and cheddar cheese and serve.

Nutrition: 119 Calories; 10 g Fats; 3.5 g Protein; 2 g Net Carb; 0.5 g Fiber;

ROASTED GREEN BEANS

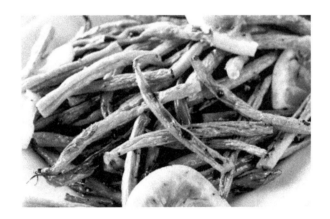

Preparation Time: 5 minutes

Cooking Time: 25 minutes;

Servings: 2

Ingredients

- ½ pound green beans
- ½ cup grated parmesan cheese
- 3 tbsp. coconut oil
- ½ tsp garlic powder
- Seasoning:
- 1/3 tsp salt
- 1/8 tsp ground black pepper

Directions:

1. Turn on the oven, then set it to 425 degrees F, and let preheat.
2. Take a baking sheet, line green beans on it, and set aside until required.

3. Prepare the dressing, and for this, place remaining ingredients in a bowl, except for cheese and whisk until combined.

4. Drizzle the dressing over green beans, toss until well coated, and then bake for 20 minutes until green beans are tender-crisp.

5. Then sprinkle cheese on top of beans and continue roasting for 3 to 5 minutes or until cheese melts and nicely golden brown.

6. Serve.

Nutrition: 119 Calories; 9 g Fats; 5 g Protein; 4.5 g Net Carb; 3 g Fiber;

FRIED CAULIFLOWER AND EGG RICE

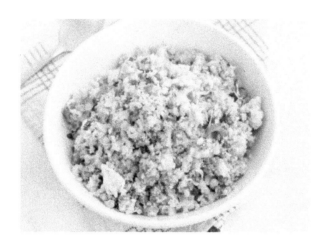

Preparation Time: 5 minutes;
Cooking Time: 12 minutes
Servings: 2
Ingredients

· 8-ounce cauliflower florets, riced
· 2 green onion, sliced
· 1 large egg, beaten
· 1 tbsp. soy sauce
· ½ tsp toasted sesame oil
· Seasoning:
· 1 tbsp. coconut oil
· ½ tsp garlic powder

Directions:

1. Take a large skillet pan, place it over medium-high heat, add coconut oil and riced cauliflower, and cook for 5 minutes until softened.
2. Then add green onions, stir well and cook for 3 minutes until onions are tender.
3. Season with salt, sprinkle garlic over cauliflower, cook for 1 minute until fragrant, then pour in the egg, stir well and cook for 2 minutes until the egg has scrambled to desire level, stirring continuously.
4. Drizzle with soy sauce and sesame oil and Serve.

Nutrition: 57 Calories; 4 g Fats; 3 g Protein; 1.7 g Net Carb; 0.5 g Fiber

SPINACH ZUCCHINI BOATS

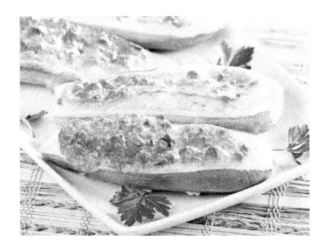

Preparation Time: 5 minutes
Cooking Time: 10 minutes;
Servings: 2
Ingredients

- 1 large zucchini
- ¾ cup spinach
- 1 ½ tbsp. whipped topping
- 3 tbsp. grated parmesan cheese
- ½ tsp garlic powder
- Seasoning:
- ½ tsp salt
- ½ tsp ground black pepper

Directions:

1. Turn on the oven, then set it to 350 degrees F, and let preheat.

2. Take a skillet pan, place it over medium heat, add spinach and cook for 5 to 7 minutes or until spinach leaves have wilted and their moisture has evaporated completely.

3. Sprinkle garlic powder, ¼ tsp each of salt and black pepper over spinach, add whipped topping and 2 tbsp. cheese and stir well until the cheese has melted, remove the pan from heat.

4. Cut off the top and bottom of zucchini, then cut it in half lengthwise and make a well by scooping out pulp along the center, leaving ½-inch shell.

5. Season zucchini with remaining salt and black pepper, place them on a baking sheet and roast for 5 minutes.

6. Then fill zucchini evenly with spinach mixture, top with remaining cheese and broil for 3 minutes until cheese has melted.

7. Serve.

Nutrition: 86.5 Calories; 6 g Fats; 4 g Protein; 3.5 g Net Carb; 0.5 g Fiber;

GREEN BEANS WITH HERBS

c

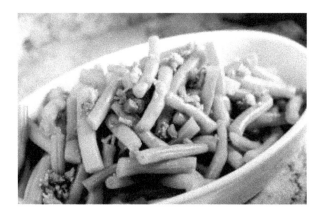

Preparation Time: 5 minutes
Cooking Time: 7 minutes;
Servings: 2
Ingredients

- 3 oz. green beans
- 2 slices of bacon, diced
- 3 tbsp. chopped parsley
- 3 tbsp. chopped cilantro
- 1 tbsp. avocado oil
- Seasoning:
- ½ tsp garlic powder
- ¼ tsp salt

Directions:

1. Place green beans in a medium heatproof bowl, cover with a plastic wrap, and then microwave for 3 to 4 minutes at high heat setting until tender.
2. Meanwhile, take a medium skillet pan, place it over medium heat and when hot, add bacon and cook for 3 to 4 minutes until crisp.
3. Season bacon with salt, sprinkle with garlic powder and cook for 30 seconds until fragrant, remove the pan from heat.
4. When green beans have steamed, drain them well, rinse under cold water, and then transfer to a bowl.
5. Add bacon and remaining ingredients and toss until well mixed.
6. Serve.

Nutrition: 380 Calories; 33.7 g Fats; 15.2 g Protein; 2.4 g Net Carb; 1.4 g Fiber;

SALAD SANDWICHES

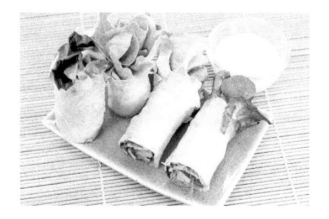

Preparation Time: 5 minutes;

Cooking Time: 0 minutes;

Servings: 2

Ingredients

- · 1 medium avocado, peeled, pitted, diced
- · 2 leaves of iceberg lettuce
- · 1-ounce unsalted butter
- · 2-ounce cheddar cheese, sliced

Directions:

1. Rinse the lettuce leaves, pat dry with a paper towel, and then smear each leaf with butter.
2. Top lettuce with cheese and avocado and serve.

Nutrition: 187 Calories; 17 g Fats; 5 g Protein; 4 g Net Carb; 1.5 g Fiber;

CELERIAC STUFFED AVOCADO

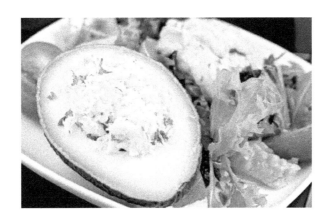

Preparation Time: 10 minutes;
Cooking Time: 0 minutes
Servings: 2
Ingredients

- · 1 avocado
- · 1 celery root, finely chopped
- · 2 tbsp. mayonnaise
- · ½ of a lemon, juiced, zested
- · 2 tbsp. mayonnaise
- · Seasoning:
- · ¼ tsp salt

Directions:

1. Prepare avocado and for this, cut avocado in half and then remove its pit.
2. Place remaining ingredients in a bowl, stir well until combined and evenly stuff this mixture into avocado halves.
3. Serve.

Nutrition: 285 Calories; 27 g Fats; 2.8 g Protein; 4.4 g Net Carb; 2.6 g Fiber;

COBB SALAD

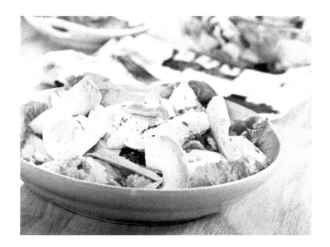

Preparation Time: 5 minutes

Cooking Time: 10 minutes;

Servings: 1

Ingredients

- · 1 large egg, hard-boiled, peeled, diced
- · 2 oz. chicken thigh
- · 2 1/2 slices bacon, cooked, crumbled
- · ½ of a medium avocado, diced
- · ½ cup chopped lettuce
- · Seasoning:
- · 1 cup of water
- · 3 tbsp. apple cider vinegar
- · 1 ½ tbsp. coconut oil
- · ¼ tsp salt
- · 1/8 tsp ground black pepper

Directions:

1. Cook chicken thigh and for this, place chicken thighs in an instant pot, pour in 1 cup water, and shut the pot with a lid.
2. Cook the chicken for 5 minutes at high pressure, and when done, let the pressure release naturally.
3. Meanwhile, cook the bacon and for this, take a skillet pan, place it over medium heat and when hot, add bacon slices.
4. Cook the bacon for 3 to 5 minutes until golden brown, then transfer them to a cutting board and chop the bacon, reserve the bacon grease in the pan for the next meal.
5. When chicken thigh has cooked, transfer it to a bowl and shred the chicken with two forks, reserving the chicken broth for later use.
6. Assemble the salad and for this, place lettuce in a salad plate, top with chicken, bacon, diced eggs, avocado, and chicken in horizontal rows.
7. Prepare the dressing and for this, whisk together salt, black pepper, vinegar, and oil until incorporated and then drizzle the dressing generously over the salad.
8. Serve.

Nutrition: 206 Calories; 11.8 g Fats; 19.2 g Protein; 6 g Net Carb; 3 g Fiber;

CHAPTER

107

CABBAGE HASH BROWNS

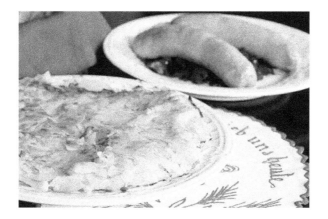

Preparation Time: 10 minutes
Cooking Time: 12 minutes
Servings: 2
Ingredients

· 1 ½ cup shredded cabbage
· 2 slices of bacon
· 1/2 tsp garlic powder
· 1 egg
· Seasoning:
· 1 tbsp. coconut oil
· ½ tsp salt
· 1/8 tsp ground black pepper

Directions:

1. Crack the egg in a bowl, add garlic powder, black pepper, and salt, whisk well, then add cabbage, toss until well mixed and shape the mixture into four patties.

2. Take a large skillet pan, place it over medium heat, add oil and when hot, add patties in it and cook for 3 minutes per side until golden brown.
3. Transfer hash browns to a plate, then add bacon into the pan and cook for 5 minutes until crispy.
4. Serve hash browns with bacon.

Nutrition: 336 Calories; 29.5 g Fats; 16 g Protein; 0.9 g Net Carb; 0.8 g Fiber;

ASPARAGUS, WITH BACON AND EGGS

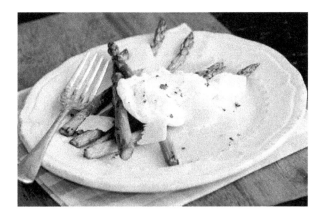

Preparation Time: 5 minutes;
Cooking Time: 12 minutes
Servings: 2
Ingredients

- · 4 oz. asparagus
- · 2 slices of bacon, diced
- · 1 egg
- · Seasoning:
- · ¼ tsp salt
- · 1/8 tsp ground black pepper

Directions:

1. Take a skillet pan, place it over medium heat, add bacon, and cook for 4 minutes until crispy.
2. Transfer cooked bacon to a plate, then add asparagus into the pan and cook for 5 minutes until tender-crisp.

3. Crack the egg over the cooked asparagus, season with salt and black pepper, then switch heat to medium-low level and cook for 2 minutes until egg white has set.
4. Chop the cooked bacon slices, sprinkle over egg and asparagus and serve.

Nutrition: 179 Calories; 15.3 g Fats; 9 g Protein; 0.7 g Net Carb; 0.6 g Fiber;

BELL PEPPER EGGS

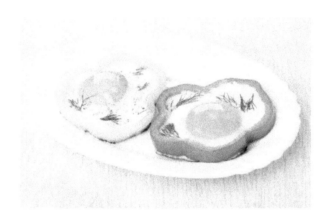

Preparation Time: 10 minutes;
Cooking Time: 4 minutes
Servings: 2
Ingredients

- · 1 green bell pepper,
- · 2 eggs
- · Seasoning:
- · 1 tsp coconut oil
- · ¼ tsp salt
- · ¼ tsp ground black pepper

Directions:

1. Prepare pepper rings, and for this, cut out two slices from the pepper, about ¼-inch, and reserve remaining bell pepper for later use.
2. Take a skillet pan, place it over medium heat, grease it with oil, place pepper rings in it, and then crack an egg into each ring.

3. Season eggs with salt and black pepper, cook for 4 minutes or until eggs have cooked to the desired level.
4. Transfer eggs to a plate and serve.

Nutrition: 110.5 Calories; 8 g Fats; 7.2 g Protein; 1.7 g Net Carb; 1.1 g Fiber;

OMELET-STUFFED PEPPERS

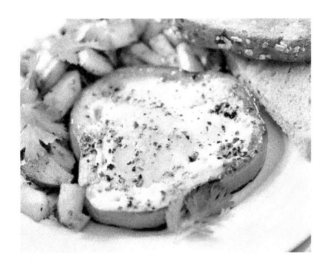

Preparation Time: 5 minutes
Cooking Time: 20 minutes
Servings: 2
Ingredients

- · 1 large green bell pepper, halved, cored
- · 2 eggs
- · 2 slices of bacon, chopped, cooked
- · 2 tbsp. grated parmesan cheese
- · Seasoning:
- · 1/3 tsp salt
- · ¼ tsp ground black pepper

Directions:

1. Turn on the oven, then set it to 400 degrees F, and let preheat.

2. Then take a baking dish, pour in 1 tbsp. water, place bell pepper halved in it, cut-side up, and bake for 5 minutes.

3. Meanwhile, crack eggs in a bowl, add chopped bacon and cheese, season with salt and black pepper, and whisk until combined.

4. After 5 minutes of baking time, remove baking dish from the oven, evenly fill the peppers with egg mixture and continue baking for 15 to 20 minutes until eggs has set.

5. Serve.

Nutrition: 428 Calories; 35.2 g Fats; 23.5 g Protein; 2.8 g Net Carb; 1.5 g Fiber;

CHAPTER

111

BACON AVOCADO BOMBS

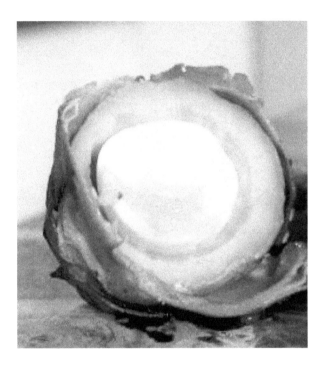

Preparation Time: 10 minutes
Cooking Time: 10 minutes
Servings: 2
Ingredients

- 1 avocado, halved, pitted
- 4 slices of bacon
- 2 tbsp. grated parmesan cheese

Directions:

1. Turn on the oven and broiler and let it preheat.

2. Meanwhile, prepare the avocado and for that, cut it in half, then remove its pit, and then peel the skin.

3. Evenly one half of the avocado with cheese, replace with the other half of avocado and then wrap avocado with bacon slices.

4. Take a baking sheet, line it with aluminum foil, place wrapped avocado on it, and broil for 5 minutes per side, flipping carefully with tong halfway.

5. When done, cut each avocado in half crosswise and serve

Nutrition: 378 Calories; 33.6 g Fats; 15.1 g Protein; 0.5 g Net Carb; 2.3 g Fiber;

EGG IN A HOLE WITH EGGPLANT

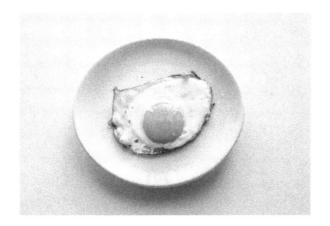

Preparation Time: 5 minutes;
Cooking Time: 15 minutes
Servings: 2
Ingredients

- · 1 large eggplant
- · 2 eggs
- · 1 tbsp. coconut oil, melted
- · 1 tsp unsalted butter
- · 2 tbsp. chopped green onions
- · Seasoning:
- · ¾ tsp ground black pepper
- · ¾ tsp salt

Directions:

1. Set the grill and let it preheat at the high setting.

2. Meanwhile, prepare the eggplant, and for this, cut two slices from eggplant, about 1-inch thick, and reserve the remaining eggplant for later use.

3. Brush slices of eggplant with oil, season with salt on both sides, then place the slices on grill and cook for 3 to 4 minutes per side.

4. Transfer grilled eggplant to a cutting board, let it cool for 5 minutes and then make a home in the center of each slice by using a cookie cutter.

5. Take a frying pan, place it over medium heat, add butter and when it melts, add eggplant slices in it and crack an egg into its each hole.

6. Let the eggs cook for 3 to 4 minutes, then carefully flip the eggplant slice and continue cooking for 3 minutes until the egg has thoroughly cooked.

7. Season egg with salt and black pepper, transfer them to a plate, then garnish with green onions and serve.

Nutrition: 184 Calories; 14.1 g Fats; 7.8 g Protein; 3 g Net Carb; 3.5 g Fiber;

FRITTATA WITH SPINACH AND MEAT

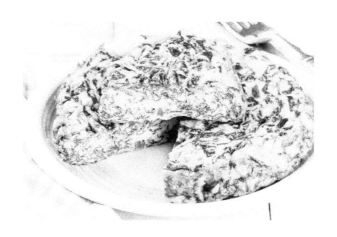

Preparation Time: 10 minutes;

Cooking Time: 20 minutes

Servings: 2

Ingredients

- · 4 oz. ground turkey
- · 3 oz. of spinach leaves
- · 1/3 tsp minced garlic
- · 1/3 tsp coconut oil
- · 2 eggs
- · Seasoning:
- · 1/3 tsp salt
- · ¼ tsp ground black pepper

Directions:

1. Turn on the oven, then set it to 400 degrees F, and let it preheat.

2. Meanwhile, take a skillet pan, place it over medium heat, and add spinach and cook for 3 to 5 minutes until spinach leaves have wilted, remove the pan from heat.

3. Take a small heatproof skillet pan, place it over medium heat, add ground turkey and cook for 5 minutes until thoroughly cooked.

4. Then add spinach, season with salt and black pepper, stir well, then remove the pan from heat and spread the mixture evenly in the pan.

5. Crack eggs in a bowl, season with salt and black pepper, then pour this mixture over spinach mixture in the pan and bake for 10 to 15 minutes until frittata has thoroughly cooked and the top is golden brown.

6. When done, let frittata rest in the pan for 5 minutes, then cut it into slices and serve.

Nutrition: 166 Calories; 13 g Fats; 10 g Protein; 0.5 g Net Carb; 0.5 g Fiber;

AVOCADO EGG BOAT WITH CHEDDAR

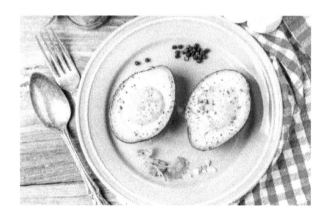

Preparation Time: 5 minutes

Cooking Time: 15 minutes

Servings: 2

Ingredients

- · 1 avocado, halved, pitted
- · 2 eggs
- · 2 tbsp. chopped bacon
- · 2 tbsp. shredded cheddar cheese
- · Seasoning:
- · 1/8 tsp salt
- · 1/8 tsp ground black pepper

Directions:

1. Turn on the oven, then set it to 400 degrees F and let it preheat.
2. Meanwhile, prepare avocado and for this, cut it into half lengthwise and then remove the pit.

3. Scoop out some of the flesh from the center, crack an egg into each half, and then sprinkle with bacon and season with salt and black pepper.
4. Sprinkle cheese over egg and avocado and then bake for 10 to 15 minutes or until the yolk has cooked to desired level.
5. Serve.

Nutrition: 263.5 Calories; 21.4 g Fats; 12 g Protein; 1.3 g Net Carb; 4.6 g Fiber

21 DAY MEAL PLAN

PlaRaspberries

Low-carb Snack List

1/4 cup: 16 calories, 0.20g fat, 3.67g carbs, 2g fiber, 0.37g protein 1/2 cup: 32 calories, 0.40g fat, 7.34g carbs, 4g fiber, 0.75g protein 1 cup: 64 calories, 0.80g fat, 14.69g carbs, 8g fiber, 1.48g protein Blueberries

1/4 cup: 21 calories, 0.12g fat, 5.25g carbs, 0.9g fiber, 0.27g protein

1/2 cup: 41 calories, 0.24g fat, 10.51g carbs, 1.7g fiber, 0.54g protein 1 cup: 83 calories, 0.48g fat, 21.01g carbs, 3.5g fiber, 1.07g protein Strawberries

1/4 cup: 12 calories, 0.11g fat, 2.92g carbs, 0.8g fiber, 0.25g protein 1/2 cup: 24 calories, 0.23g fat, 5.84g carbs, 1.5g fiber, 0.51g protein 1cup: 49 calories, 0.46g fat, 11.67g carbs, 3g fiber, 1.07g protein

Blackberries

1/4 cup: 15 calories, 0.18g fat, 3.46g carbs, 1.9g fiber, 0.5g protein 1/2 cup: 31 calories, 0.35g fat, 6.92g carbs, 3.8g fiber, 1g protein 1cup: 62 calories, 0.71g fat, 13.84g carbs, 7.6g fiber, 2g protein Nuts (Raw)

Almonds

1/4 cup: 160 calories, 14g fat, 6g carbs, 4g fiber, 6g protein

Cashews

1/4 cup: 160 calories, 12g fat, 8g carbs, 1g fiber, 5g protein Pecans

1/4 cup: 210 calories, 21g fat, 4g carbs, 2g fiber, 3g protein

Walnuts

1/4 cup: 190 calories, 18g fat, 4g carbs, 2g fiber, 4g protein Boiled Egg

1egg: 78 calories, 5.3g fat, 0.56g carbs, 0g fiber, 6.29g protein

Avocado

1/2 fruit: 161 calories, 14.73g fat, 8.57g carbs, 6.7g fiber, 2.01g protein Kalamata Olives

10 olives: 90 calories, 9g fat, 2g carbs, 2g fiber, 2g protein Almond Nut Butter

2 tbsp: 190 calories, 18g fat, 6g carbs, 3g fiber, 7g protein

Peeled Cucumber

1cup: 16 calories, 0.21g fat, 2.87g carbs, 2.8g fiber, 0.78g protein Celery Sticks

2 sticks: 15 calories, 0g fat, 4g carbs, 2g fiber, 1g protein

The following snack ideas depend on the brand or preparation method. Deviled Egg Can of tuna

Cold meat —Leftover from a roast or deli meat like ham, salami, chicken, beef, etc.

CHAPTER

116

WEEK 1 MENU

	Breakfast	Lunch ·	Dinner	Nutritional Info
Day 1	Avocado Bun Breakfast Burger	Avocado Cream & Zoodles	Chicken Cutlet and Cauli Rice	1765 calories 139.05g fat 20.75g net carbs 12.16g sugars 90.91g protein
Day 2	Breakfast Sausage, Eggs & Greens	Chicken Cutlet & Cauli Rice Leftovers	Shirataki Noodles Asian Salad	1374 calories 93g fat 19.79g net carbs 12.35g sugars 98.61g protein
Day 3	Breakfast Sausage & Eggs	BLT Lettuce Boats	Grilled Cod & Shrimps	1177calories 78.94g fat 15.74g net carbs 6.92g sugars 94.65g net carbs
Day 4	90 sec Sausage Egg Muffin	Grilled Cod & Shrimps Leftovers	Arugula Caesar Salad & Veggies	1316 calories 89g fat 19.75g net carbs 11.92g sugars 99.06g protein
Day 5	Breakfast Sausage& Poached Egg	Rosemary Chicken & Broccoli	Rosemary Pork Roast Leftovers Side Caesar Salad 3	1495 calories 111.31gfat 12.34g net carbs 7.29g sugars 101.2g protein
Day 6	Spinach & Breakfast Sausage Omelette	Rosemary Pork Roast Leftovers Side Caesar Salad 2	Broccoli, Bacon & Mushrooms	1313 calories 99.55g fat 13.02g net carbs 9.71g sugars 84.98g protein
Day 7 6	Spinach & Pork Omelette Leftovers	Zucchini Salad with Grilled Chicken Thigh	Rosemary Pork Roast Leftovers Side Caesar Salad 1	1509 calories 114.98g fat 15.62g net carbs 10.28g sugars 96.37g protein

WEEK 1 GROCERY LIST

Baking
Baking Powder [1/2 tsp]
Blanched Almond Flour [7 tbsp]
Pork Rinds [40g]
Condiments
Anchovy Paste [10 ml]
Coconus Aminos [25 ml]
Fish Sauce [5 ml]
Lemon Juice [25 ml]
Mayonnaise [125 ml]
White Vinegar [20 ml]
Dairy
Almond Milk [45ml]
Eggs [19]
Meat
Bacon [5 slices]
Chicken Breast [1] {260g}skinless
Chicken Thighs [3] {200g} boneless
Ground Chicken [220g]
Ground Pork [220g]
Pork Roast Boneless [500g]
Prosciutto [60g]
Oil
Chili Oil [1/4 tsp](orcayenne pepper)
Frying Oil (Could be refined coconut oil, lard orbeef tallow)
Olive oil [215ml]
Refined Coconut Oil [15ml]
Sesame Oil [35ml]

Seafood & Fish

Cod Fillets [2] {300g}

Shrimps [200g]

Spices

Black Pepper

Cayenne Pepper

Celery Seed

Dashi Powder (Japanese Fish Broth Granule)

Garlic Powder

Himalayan Salt

Nutmeg

Onion Powder

Oregano

Paprika Powder

Parsley

Rosemary

Sage

Sesame Seeds

Thyme

Vegetables

Arugula [40g]

Asparagus [6 stems] {120g}

Avocado [2 3/4 hass]

Baby Spinach [2 cups] {80g}

Basil Leaves [25 leaves]

Broccoli [3 heads]

Brown Mushrooms [7]{70g}

Cauliflower [1 small]{300g}

Cherry Tomatoes [14]

Cilantro [1 stem]

Cucumber [3/4 cup] {85g}

Garlic [9 cloves]

Green Beans[50g]

Lettuce [18 leaves]

Parsley [2 stems]

Red Onion [1/16]

Red Pepper [3/4]

Swiss Chard [50g]

Tomato [4]

Zucchini [1 1/4]

Miscellaneous
Shirataki Noodles [200g]

WEEK 1

Day 1 - Make Ahead

1. **Savoury Breakfast Sausage**

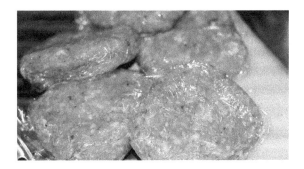

185 calories 12.81g fat0.25g carbs0.2g fiber0.04g sugar16.17g protein

Mix all of the ingredients in a bowl and knead with
your hands.

Make six hamburger patty, wrap them in saran wrap and freeze them. We'll be using these for the next 6 days so if you think the meat will stay fresh, you don't have to freeze them, but I did just in case. I just thaw each hamburger the night before or thaw them in the microwave the day of.

Ingredients (6 portions) 220g ground chicken 220g ground pork

1tsp sage

1/2 tsp salt, thyme, black pepper 1/4 tsp celery seed, garlic powder, nutmeg, onion powder, paprika 1/8 tsp cayenne pepper

Day 1 - Breakfast

2. **Avocado Bun Breakfast Burger**

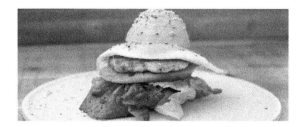

717 calories61.36g fat20.11g carbs 14.6g fiber2.88g sugar27.41g protein

Lay the avocado on its side, horizontally, and cut it right in the middle making sure you're not cutting it in an awkward angle. Once it 's cut, carefully re- move the seed and carefully spoon out of the flesh. Cut the bottom of one avocado so that it can stand on its own on the plate.

Heat the oil in a non-stick skillet on medium-low heat. Add the breakfast sausage and cook 1-2 min- utes on each side until perfectly cooked. Crack the egg open in the skillet, turn the heat to low, cover and cook sunny side up. Cook for a couple of min- utes until the egg white is fully cooked.

Place the bottom half of the avocado on a plate, spoon some mayo in the avocado hole, top with lettuce, the tomato, sausage, carefully add the egg over and top wth the avocado top! Sprinkle some salt, pepper and sesame seeds.

Ingredients (1 portion)

1 avocado

1 egg

1tbsp olive oil 1breakfast sausage 1lettuce leaf

1slice tomato

1tbsp mayo

pinch salt, pepper, sesame seeds

3. **Avocado Cream & Zoodles**

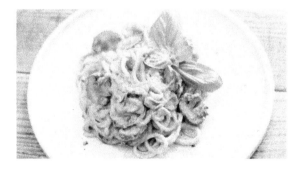

383 calories 35.34g fat18g carbs9.4g fiber4.74g sugar5.46g protein

Spiralize your zucchini. Slice the mushrooms in
half.

In a stick blender cup, add the avocado, basil, 1tbsp olive oil, garlic, lemon juice and salt. Press the but- ton on the stick blender for about a minute until everything is su- per creamy and delicious.

Add 1/2 tbsp of olive oil in a frying pan and cook the mushrooms until tender. Add the zucchini noodles and cook just for a minute or so until they get hot.

Add the avocado cream, mix everything together

and serve.

Ingredients (1 portion)

1 zucchini

1/2 avocado (100g) 20 basil leaves

1.5 tbsp olive oil

3 brown mushrooms (30g) 1garlic clove

1tsp lemon juice 1/4 tsp salt

4. **Chicken Cutlet & CauliRice**

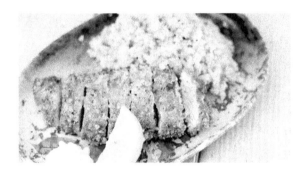

665 calories 42.35g fat14.64g carbs 8g fiber54. g sugar58.04g protein

Ingredients (2 portions)

Rice the cauliflower in a food processor or by using a cheese grater. In a wok, heat the sesame oil and add the riced cauliflower. Fry a couple of minutes, add the coconut aminos, dashi, salt and pepper, and mix until combined. Fry until the cauliflower is soft and crunchy.

Crush the pork rinds using a food processor/coffee grinder/or your hands. Mix the rinds with the al- mond flour, salt and pepper. Add the egg in a small bowl and whisk. Slice the chicken breast in 2 lenght ways. Sprinkle the salt and pepper on both sides and dip in it the whisked egg. Coat the chicken with the breading on both sides.

Fry the cutlet in 150C/300F preheated oil and fry until the inner temperature of the chciken cutlet registers to 65C/150F. Serve with the cauli rice. Keep half for another meal.

small cauliflower (300g)

tbsp sesame oil 1tbsp coconut aminos 1tsp dashi powder

1/4 tsp salt + pepper

1skinless chicken breast (260g)

pinch salt + pepper

1 egg

4 tbsp almond flour 40g pork rinds pinch salt + pepper

frying oil (refined coconut oil/lard/ beef tallow)

5. **Breakfast Sausage, Eggs & Greens**

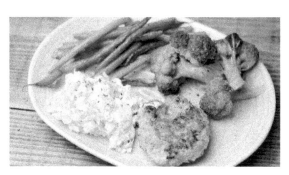

560 calories 43.30g fat12g carbs7g fiber2.79g sugar31.71g protein

Cut the stems off the green beans. Mince the gar-lic.

Put some water to boil in a pot. Add the broccoli and green beans and cook until tender. Take out of the water once cooked. Place the broccoli onto a plate.

Add the olive oil to a frying pan and add the break- fast sausage. Cook on both sides until cooked through. Add the eggs and scramble them. Place the eggs and sausage to the plate.

Add the garlic and green beans to the frying pan.

Fry until the garlic is starting to crisp up. Sprinkle some salt, pepper and garlic powder over the beans and scrambled eggs. Place the beans and eggs onto the plate.

Ingredients (1 portion)

breakfast sausage

eggs

4 broccoli florets 50g green beans

1.5 tbsp olive oil 1garlic clove

pinch salt, pepper, garlic powder

6. **Chicken Cutlet & CauliRice**

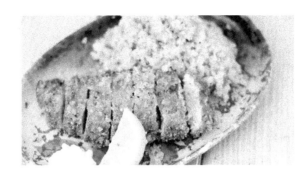

665 calories 42.35g fat14.64g carbs 8g fiber4.54g sugar58.04g protein

Ingredients (2 portions)

1. Heat up the leftovers from last night's dinner!

2nd portion of Day 1 dinner!

7. Shirataki Noodles Asian Salad

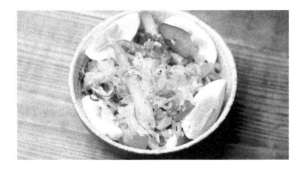

149 calories 7.53g fat12.45g carbs 4.3g fiber5.02g sugar8.86g protein

Put some water to boil in a pot. Place the egg in- side and boil for 7 minutes exactly. Once cooked, transfer to a bowl full of ice water. Peel and cut in four.

Wash the shirataki noodles under some water and boil for 2 minutes. This will get rid of their smell. In the same pot, add the asparagus and boil until tender. Drain the water and let the noodles and

asparagus cool down. You can cut the noodles in half to make them shorter as they tend to be super long.

Thinly slice the red onion with a cabbage shredder. Cut the asparagus in half. Dice the tomato, slice the cucumber, chop the cilantro, and mince the

garlic using a garlic crusher.

Combine all of the ingredients in a large bowl and

mix. Serve cold!

Ingredients (1 portion)

200 g shirataki noodles (konjac) 2 asparagus (40g)

1/2 cup cucumber (65g)

1/2 tomato (65g) 1/16 red onions (20g) 1stem cilantro

1 garlic

egg

2tsp coconut aminos

1tsp fish sauce 1/2 tsp sesame oil 1tsp lemon juice

1/4 tsp salt and pepper

8. Breakfast Sausage & Eggs

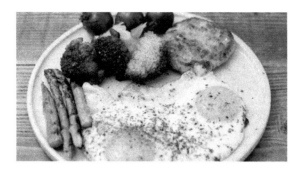

477 calories 36.51g fat6.40g carbs2.5g fiber3.16g sugar30.61g protein

Cut the asparagus in two and cut off a bit off the

stems.

Put some water to boil and add the broccoli. Cook until tender.

Add 1/2 tbsp of olive oil to a non-stick frying pan and add the breakfast sausage and asparagus and cook on all sides until cooked through. Transfer to a plate with the boiled broccoli.

Add the other 1/2 tbsp of olive oil and crack the

eggs open. Switch the heat to low, cover and cook for a few minutes until the egg whites are fully cooked. Slide to the plate and sprinkle the salt, pepper and parsley over.

Ingredients (1 portion)

eggs

1breakfast sausage 1tbsp olive oil

asparagus

broccoli

3 cherry tomatoes

pinch salt, pepper, parsley

9. BLT Lettuce Boats

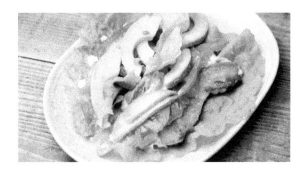

362 calories 33.20g fat10.64g carbs 3.34g fiber1.79g sugar8.62g protein

Fry the bacon in a frying pan until crispy.

Slice the tomato into a few slices. Slice the avocado.

Spoon 1/2 tbsp of mayo over each lettuce leaf and cover with the bacon, tomato and avocado.

Ingredients (1 portion)

2 lettuce leaves

2 slices bacon 1/2 avocado 1/4 tomato

1tbsp mayo

10. **Grilled Cod & Shrimps**

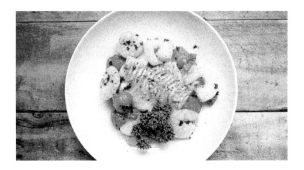

338 calories 9.23g fat5.54g carbs1g fiber1.97g sugar55.42g protein

Mince the garlic and parsley

Melt the butter in a pan and add the garlic. Cook for a few seconds and place the cod and shrimp in the pan. Add the chopped parsley. Cook the shrimps for a few minutes until they turn orange. For the cod, cook for 2 minutes on each side, carefully not breaking it apart when flipping it over. Add the

tomatoes to the pan and fry with the shrimps for about a minute until soft.

Add the lemon juice over everything and it 's ready

to serve. Store half for tomorrow.

Ingredients (2 portions) 2 cod fillet (300g)

200g shrimps

tbsp lemon juice 2stems fresh parsley 2 tbsp olive oil

garlic cloves

8 cherry toamtoes

11. **Easy Dairy-free CaesarDressing**

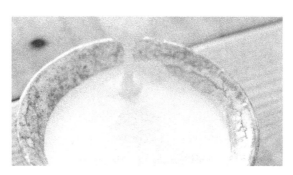

106 calories 11.39g fat0.4g carbs0.1g fiber0.02g sugar0.32g protein

1. Mince the garlic. Mix all of the ingredients together

and keep in an air-tight container in the fridge. It will keep for weeks, just mix it again before using.

Ingredients (6 portions)

6 tbsp mayonnaise 2tsp anchovy paste 1garlic clove

3tbsp unsweetened almond milk 1/2 tsp lemon juice

1.5 tsp oregano 1/8 tsp salt

1/4 tsp garlic powder

12. **9 0 sec Sausage Egg McMuffin**

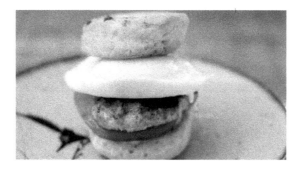

719 calories60.15g fat9.38g carbs4.15g fiber2.61g sugar36.57g protein

Combine the ingredients for the 90 second bread into a large mug. Mix carefully and microwave for 90 seconds. Take it out of the mug and carefully

slice in half.

Heat the olive oil in a frying pan and fry the break- fast sausage until cooked. Add the sliced bread and grill on both sides until desired toastness.

Using a mini egg frying pan, cook the egg until the

egg whites are fully cooked.

Spread the mayo over one slice of bread, cover with the tomato slice, sausage, egg and last slice of bread. Enjoy!!

Ingredients (1 portion) 1breakfast sausage 1slice tomato

1 egg

1tsp olive oil 1tsp mayo

90 sec bread: mix all of these

*1 tbsp refined coconut oil

*1 egg

*1/2 tsp salt

*1/2 tsp baking powder

*3 tbsp almond flour

13. **Grilled Cod & Shrimps**

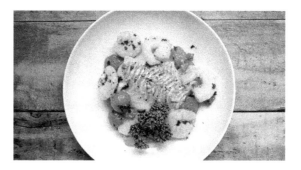

338 calories 9.23g fat5.54g carbs1g fiber1.97g sugar55.42g protein

1. Reheat yesterday's dinners leftover and enjoy!

Ingredients (2 portions) Leftovers from Day 3 Dinner

14. **Arugula Caesar Salad & Veggies**

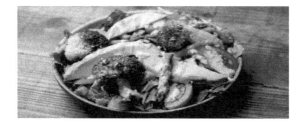

259 calories 19.62g fat19.08g carbs 9.1g fiber7.34g sugar7.07g protein

Put some water to boil and cook the broccoli and

asparagus until tender.

Shred the ruccola and iceberg lettuce and put into a bowl.

Slice the avocado, tomato, and cucumber. Put ev-

erything in a plate and cover with the dressing.

Ingredients (1 portion)

3 leaves iceberg lettuce (120g) 40g arugula

2 asparagus (60g)

4 broccoli florets (60g)

5-6 slices cucumber (20g)

1/2 avocado

1/2 tomato

1portion caesar dressing

15. Breakfast Sausage & Poached Egg

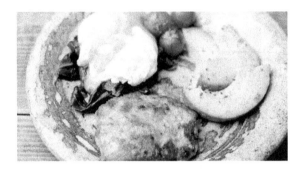

461 calories 37.54g fat7.08g carbs4.2g fiber1.93g sugar24.55g protein

Put some water to heat in a small pot and add the vinegar. Crack the egg inside a small bowl or cup. Once the water is simmering, make a circulating motion with a spatula inside the water and drop the egg in the middle of the spiral. Turn off the heat, cover for 6 minutes exactly. Take it out of the water once done.

Heat the olive oil in a frying pan and cook the breakfast sausage on medium-low heat on both sides until cooked through. Place the sausage on a plate. Add the fresh spinach to the frying pan with the leftover grease from the sausage. Cook

until wilted and transfer to a plate. Cover with the poached egg.

Slice the avocado and put on the plate along with the cherry tomatoes.

Ingredients (1 portion) 1breakfast sausage 1tbsp olive oil

egg

40g fresh spinach 3 cherry tomatoes 1/4 avocado

1/4 tsp salt & pepper 1tbsp vinegar

16. Rosemary Chicken & Broccoli

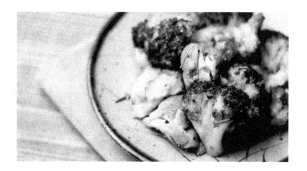

461 calories 33.71g fat6.99g carbs2.8g fiber1.7g sugar33.94g protein

Cut the chicken leg into bite-size pieces. Sprinkle the salt and pepper all over it. Separate the broccoli into florets.

In a cast iron skillet, heat the olive oil and add the chicken skin side down to the pan along with the rosemary. Fry 3 minutes to crisp up the skin and turn the chicken around. Add the broccoli florets and cook for a minute mixing everything together. Add the water, cover and let the steam of the water cook the broccoli for 2 minutes. Uncover and serve.

Ingredients (1 portion) 1boneless chicken leg (125g) 1/3 broccoli head (100g)

1/4 tsp salt

1/4 tsp black pepper 1/2 tsp rosemary 1tbsp olive oil

tbsp water

17. Rosemary Pork Roast

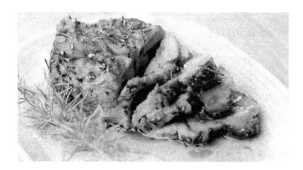

359 calories 23.88g fat0.12g carbs0.1g fiber0g sugar 33.75g protein

Preheat the oven to 200C/400F.

Massage the olive oil, salt, black pepper and rose- mary into the pork roast. Place it on a baking tray over some parchment paper.

Place in the oven and cook 1hour. Take it out and let cool for 5-10 minutes. Slice and serve. Keep 2/3 for the other meals.

Ingredients (3 portions) 500g boneless pork roast 1tbsp olive oil

1tsp salt

1tsp black pepper

1tbsp rosemary

18. Side Caesar Salad 3

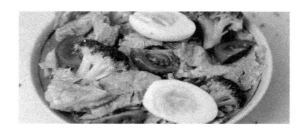

214 calories 16.72g fat 7.85g carbs 2.6g fiber 3.66g sugar 8.96g protein

Put some water to boil and add the egg. Boil for 7 minutes exactly, transfer to an bowl filled with ice water. Peel it. Put the broccoli to boil and cook until tender.

Slice the broccoli and egg. Rip the lettuce leaves.

Mix everything together with the caesar dress- ing and eat with one portion of the rosemary pork roast.

Ingredients (1 portion)

4 lettuce leaves

1 egg

1/2 tomato

3 broccoli stems (50g)

1tbsp caesar dressing

19. Spinach & Pork Omelette

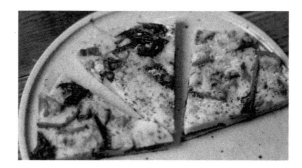

446 calories 34.96g fat 4.29g carbs 0.9g fiber 3.39g sugar 27.84g protein

Crumble the sausage. Slice the red pepper and

mince the garlic.

In a large non-stick frying pan, add the olive oil and cook the sausage. Add the garlic, red pepper and

spinach to the pan and cook for 1-2 minutes until

soft.

Crack the eggs open in a large bowl, add the spices and mix with a whisk for 2 minutes.

Pour the egg batter to the pan, cover and let cook on low heat for 4-5 minutes.

When the top of the omeltte is cooked through, just slide the omelette to a plate and cut in half. Save half for the next day.

Ingredients (2 portions) 1breakfast sausage 1cup fresh spinach (30g)

1/4 red pepper (40g) 2garlic cloves

2 tbsp olive oil

1/4 tsp salt, pepper, garlic powder, parsley

6 eggs

20. **Rosemary Pork Roast**

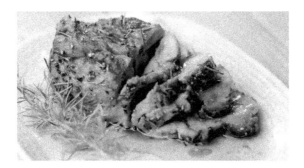

359 calories 23.88g fat0.12g carbs0.1g fiber0g sugar33.75g protein

1. Reheat 1/3 of the pork roast from Day 5 dinner.

Ingredients (3 portions) Leftovers from Dinner 5 Dinner

21. **Side Caesar Salad2**

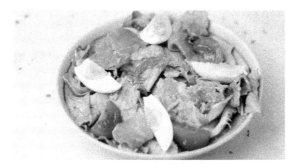

264 calories 19.15 fat6.64g carbs2g fiber4.19g sugar16.32g protein

Put some water to boil and add the egg. Boil for 7 minutes exactly, transfer to an bowl filled with ice water. Peel it.

Slice the egg in four. Rip the lettuce leaves.

Mix everything together with the caesar dressing and eat with the leftover pork roast.

Ingredients (1 portion)

4 lettuce leaves 30g prosciutto 1 egg

1 tomato

1tbsp caesar dressing

22. **Bacon, Broccoli & Mushrooms**

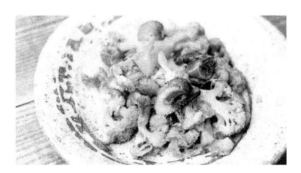

386 calories 26.22g fat4g carbs1.6g fiber0.98g sugar32.72g protein

Put some water to boil in a small pot and cook the

broccoli until tender.

Sprinkle the salt over the bacon slices and cut into 1cm strips.

Cut the mushrooms in 6.

Fry the bacon in a frying pan for a minute and add the mushrooms. Add the rosemary and fry until the bacon is crispy. Add the broccoli, mix everything together and sprinkle the garlic podwer and black pepper over.

Ingredients (1 portion) 80g broccoli

brown mushrooms (40g) 3 slices bacon (40g cooked) 1/4 tsp salt

1/2 tsp rosemary

1/4 tsp garlic powder pinch black pepper.

23. **Spinach & Pork Omelette**

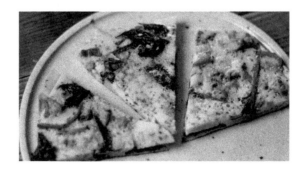

446 calories 34.96g fat4.29g carbs0.9g fiber3.39g sugar27.84g protein

1. Reheat Day 6's breakfast leftovers.Ingredients (2 portions)

leftovers from Day 6 breakfast

24. **Zucchini Salad w/ Grilled Chicken Thigh**

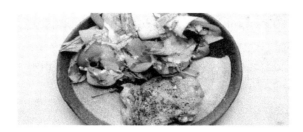

430 calories 36.93g fat8.18g carbs2.6g fiber3.89g sugar17.84g protein

Using a peeler, peel the zucchini lenghtwise to

make long ribbons. Slice the red pepper and cut in half. Dice the tomato. Chop the swiss chard. Mince the basil leaves and garlic cloves.

Mix all of the above with the olive oil, vinegar and

salt & pepper together in a bowl and put on a plate.

Sprinkle the salt and pepper over the chicken thigh. Preheat the oil in a cast iron skillet and place chicken breast skin-side down and cook until crispy. Turn it around, cook a few more minutes until cooked through. Place on the plate with the salad.

Ingredients (1 portion)

1/4 zucchini

1/4 red pepper 50g swiss chard 1/4 tomato

basil leaves 1tbsp olive oil 1tsp vinegar

1 garlic clove

1/4 tsp salt & pepper

1chicken thigh with skin (75g) 1tbsp olive oil

1/2 tsp salt & pepper

25. **Rosemary Pork Roast**

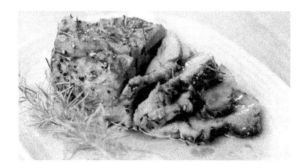

359 calories 23.88g fat0.12g carbs0.1g fiber0g sugar33.75g protein

1. Reheat the leftovers from Day 5's dinner and serve

with the side caesar salad 1.

Ingredients (3 portions) leftovers from Day 5 Dinner

26. **Side Caesar Salad1**

274 calories 19.21g fat8.83g carbs2.2g fiber3g sugar16.94g protein

Put some water to boil and add the egg. Boil for 7 minutes exactly, transfer to an bowl filled with ice water. Peel it. Put the broccoli to boil and cook until tender.

Slice the broccoli and egg. Rip the lettuce leaves.

Slice the tomato and red pepper.

Mix everything together with the caesar dress- ing and eat with one portion of the rosemary pork roast.

Ingredients (1 portion)

4 lettuce leaves 30g prosciutto 1 egg

1/2 tomato

1/4 red pepper

2 broccoli stems (25g)

1tbsp caesar dressing

WEEK 2 MENU

	Breakfast	Lunch	Dinner	Nutritional Info
Day 8	Avocado Boat, Sausage & Asparagus	Rosemary Shrimps & Radishes	Chicken Brochettes and Sesame Salad	1266 calories 91.45g fat 16.02g net carbs 8.52g sugars 81.77g protein
Day 9	Eggs, Bacon & Tomato Salad	Chicken Brochettes & Easy Sesame Salad	Lettuce-wrapped Burger	1299 calories 97.34g fat 16.86g net carbs 11.5g sugars 80.22g protein
Day 10	Avocado Boat, Sausages, & Scrambled Eggs	Chicken Bro- chettes & Sesame Salad	Arugula Salad with Basil Vinaigrette	1529 calories 120.89g fat 19.48g net carbs 10.59g sugars 40.37g protein
Day 11	Fluffy Omelette & Veggies	Zucchini & Cucumber Salad	Roasted Chicken Leg & Veggies	1191 calories 83g fat 19.08g net carbs 13.48g sugars 85.18g protein
Day 12	Grilled Veggies & Fluffy Omelette	Roasted Chicken Leg & Veggies Leftovers	Cauliflower & Veggie Ranch Salad	1434 calories 103.26g fat 19.79g net carbs 14.77g sugars 97.3g protein
Day 13	Veggie Omelette	Kale Beef & Veggie Caesar Wrap	Grilled Rosemary Chicken with Veggies	1779calories 125.69g fat 20.33g net carbs 9.46g sugars 92.39g protein
Day 14 34	Eggs in Mini Skillet	Grilled Rosemary Chicken with Veggies Leftovers	Grilled Chicken & Guacamole	1834 calories 130.48g fat 17.71gnet carbs 9.11g sugars 95.34g protein

WEEK 2 GROCERY LIST

Canned Goods

Tuna [140g]

Condiments

Coconut Aminos [37 ml]

Lemon Juice [15 ml]

Mayonnaise [112 ml]

Tahini [15 ml] (sesamepaste)

White Vinegar [20 ml]

Dairy

Almond Milk Unsweetened [5 ml]

Eggs [14]

Fruits

Lemon [2]

Meat

Bacon [7 slices]

Breakfast Pork Sausage [5] {200g}

Chicken Leg [4] {1100g} boneless

Chicken Leg [2] {600g} bone-in

Chicken Thigh [1] {150g} withskin

Ground Beef [70g]

Prosciutto [60g]

Thinly Sliced Beef[100g]

Oil

Chili Oil [1/4tsp]

Olive Oil [205 ml]

Sesame Oil [15 ml]

Spices

Black Pepper

Chili Powder

Cumin Powder

Garlic Powder

Himalayan Salt

Onion Powder

Oregano

Paprika Powder

Parsley

Rosemary

Sesame Seeds

Stevia Powder [1/16 tsp]

Thyme

Vegetables

Arugula [40g]

Asparagus [12 stems] {320g}

Avocado [3 hass]

Basil Leaves [11]

Black Olives [2 tbsp]

Brown Mushrooms [10]

Broccoli [2 heads]

Cauliflower [3 florets]

Cherry Tomatoes [18 cherries]

Cucumber [1 cup]

Garlic [16]

Kale [1 leaf] {50g}

Lettuce [16 leaves]

Long Asian Green Onion [1] (JapaneseLeek)

Mini Carrots [1 bag] (about200g)

Okra [2]

Radishes [15]

Red Onion [1/2]

Red Pepper [1 1/2]

Spinach [4 1/4 cups]

Spring Onions [2 stems]

Swiss Chard [30g]

Tomato [4]

Zucchini [1 1/2]

WEEK 2

Day 8 - Breakfast

1. **Avocado Boat, Sausage & Asparagus**

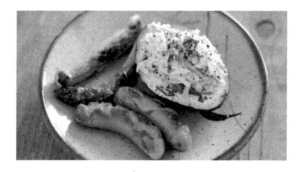

537 calories 42.29g fat11.2g carbs8.3g fiber1.3g sugar30.78g protein
Heat the olive oil in a small frying pan and fry the sausages and asparagus until cooked through. Transfer to a plate.
Scoop the inside of the avocado and place it in a bowl, along with the tuna, wilted spinach, mayo and salt & pepper. Stuff the avocado shell with it and place on the plate.
Ingredients (1 portion) 60g sausage
1-2 asparagus 1tsp olive oil 1/2 avocado 70g tuna
1/4 cup wilted spinach (50g fresh) 1tbsp mayo
pinch salt & pepper

Day 8 - Lunch
2. **Rosemary Shrimps & Radishes**

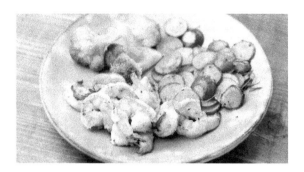

261 calories15.63g fat8.13g carbs3.2g fiber2.82g sugar22.64g protein

Put some water to boil in a pot and add the broccoli. Cook until tender.

In a skillet, heat the oil and add the radishes to one side and the shrimps to another.

Sprinkle the salt, pepper and rosemary and cook for a few minutes.

The radishes should be soft and crunchy, and the

shrimps should be orange.

Put everything on a plate and enjoy!

Ingredients (1 portion)

5 radishes (85g)

10 shrimps (100g)

3 broccoli florets (60g) 1tbsp rosemary

1tbsp olive oil

1/2 tsp salt, pepper

3. Soy & Dairy-free Creamy Sesame Dressing

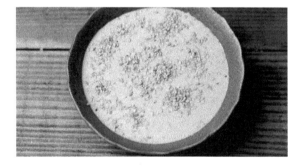

61 calories5.95g fat1.27g carbs1g fiber0g sugar0.42g protein

1. Mix all of the ingredients together in a small bowl. Store in an air-tight container in the fridge. Just remix with a spoon before use each time.

Ingredients (10 portions)

3 tbsp mayo

2.5 tbsp coconut aminos 1tbsp sesame oil

1tbsp tahini

1tbsp crushed sesame seeds 1tbsp sesame seeds

1tsp vinegar

1/16 tsp stevia powder

4. Chicken & VegetableBrochettes

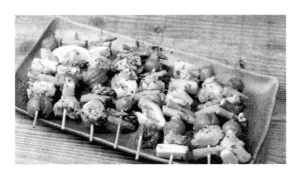

317 calories20.11g fat7.21g carbs1.5g fiber2.79g sugar26.35g protein

Preheat the oven to 210C/420F.

Dice the chicken leg into bite size pieces. Slice the long green onion into 12-14 pieces. Cut the aspara- gus into 4.

Add all of the ingredients to a bowl and mix togeth- er. Skewer the veggies and chicken on 9 brochettes.

Place in the oven and bake for 20 minutes.

Ingredients (3 portions) 1boneless chicken leg (300g) 4 asparagus

1large asian green onion

1tbsp lemon juice from a lemon 1tbsp rosemary

10 cherry tomatoes 1tbsp olive oil 1tsp salt & pepper 5 garlic cloves

1/2 tsp onion powder

5. Chicken Brochettes & SesameSalad

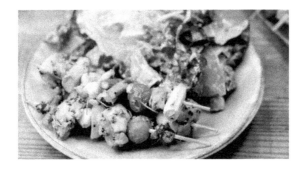

468 calories 33.53g fat14.89g carbs 6.7g fiber4.44g sugar28.35g protein

Rip the lettuce into bite size pieces. Scoop out the avocado and cube it, slice the tomato slice in a few pieces. Add the sesame dressing and coat well.

Add the brochettes to a plate along with the salad.

Ingredients (1 portion)

3 chicken & veggie brochettes 3 lettuce leaves

1tomato slice

1/4 avocado

1portion sesame dressing

6. **Eggs, Bacon & Tomato Salad**

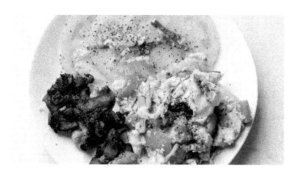

541 calories 39.81g fat8.12g carbs1.8g fiber4.42g sugar36.3g protein

Slice the red pepper and zucchini.

Fry the bacon in a small non-stick frying pan until crispy. Put the bacon on a plate. Fry the peppers and zucchini in the bacon fat until tender, crack the eggs open and scramble until cooked. Sprinkle the salt and pepper over. Put on the plate with the bacon.

Mince the garlic clove and basil leaf. Mix the olive oil, basil, garlic, vinegar, salt & pepper together in a small bowl. Add the tomato slices to the plate and pour the dressing over.

Ingredients (1 portion)

3 slices bacon

eggs

1/4 red pepper 1/4 zucchini (40g)

pinch salt & pepper

slices tomato

1basil leaf 1tsp olive oil 1garlic clove

1/2 tsp vinegar

sprinkle salt & pepper

7. **Chicken Brochettes & Easy Salad**

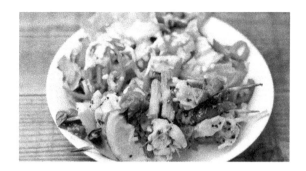

400 calories 26.29g fat13.28g carbs 4.2g fiber5.89g sugar27.92g protein

Rip the lettuce into bite size pieces. Slice the red pepper and tomato. Add the sesame dressing and coat well.

Add the brochettes to a plate along with the salad.

Ingredients (1 portion)

3 chicken brochettes

5 lettuce leaves 1/4 red pepper 1slice tomato

1tbsp sesame dressing

8. Lettuce-wrapped Burger

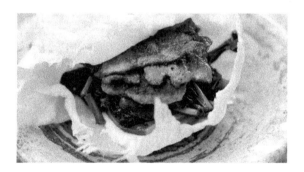

358 calories 31.24g fat2.76g carbs1.3g fiber1.19g sugar16g protein

Fry the bacon in a skillet until crispy. Form a ham- burger patty with the ground beef and fry in the leftover bacon grease. Cook on both sides until cooked through.

Add the spinach to the leftover grease in the skillet and cook until wilted.

Add the mayo, tomato, spinach, patty and bacon in

a large lettuce leaf, fold and make a burger!

Ingredients (1 portion)

70g ground beef

slices bacon (50g) (18g cooked) 1large lettuce leaf

1cup fresh baby spinach

9. 1slice tomato 1tbsp mayo

10. Basil Vinaigrette

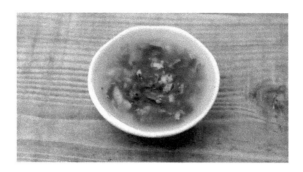

188 calories 20.28g fat2.27g carbs0.2g fiber0.24g sugar0.38g protein

1. Crush the garlic cloves using a garlic crusher. Mince the basil leaves. Combine all of the ingre- dients into a bowl and mix. Refrigerate until later used.

Ingredients (2 portions) 3 tbsp olive oil

1tbsp white vinegar 1tbsp lemon juice

garlic cloves

10 basil leaves

1/4 tsp salt, pepper

11. Avocado Boat, Sausages & Scrambled Eggs

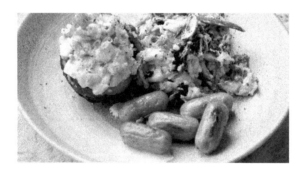

792 calories 64.82g fat11.23g carbs 7.5g fiber2.19g sugar42.93g protein

Slice the mushrooms.

Heat the oil in a small non stick frying pan and fry the sausages. Once cooked, add them to a plate. Fry the mushrooms and fresh spinach until soft and add the eggs. Scramble until cooked, sprinkle the

salt and pepper, and add to the plate.

Scoop out the insides of the avocado, and mix with the green onions, tuna, mayo and salt and pepper in a small bowl. Refill the avocado shell with the bowl ingredients and place on the plate.

Ingredients (1 portion)

60g sausage

2 eggs

mushrooms 1/4 spinach 1tbsp olive oil

pinch salt & pepper 1/2 avocado

70g tuna can

1tbsp mayo

1tsp sliced green onion pinch salt & pepper

12. **Chicken Brochettes & SesameSalad**

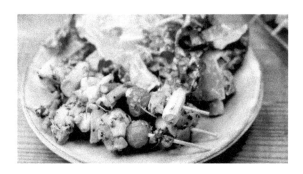

468 calories 33.53g fat14.89g carbs 6.7g fiber4.44g sugar28.35g protein

Rip the lettuce into bite size pieces. Scoop out the avocado and cube it, slice the tomato slice in a few pieces. Add the sesame dressing and coat well.

Add the brochettes to a plate along with the salad.

Ingredients (1 portion)

chicken & veggie brochettes 3 lettuce leaves

1tomato slice

1/4 avocado

1tbsp sesame dressing

13. **Arugula salad with Basil Vinaigrette**

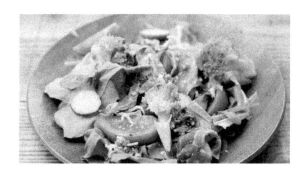

269 calories 22.54g fat10.46g carbs 2.9g fiber3.96g sugar9.09g protein

Put some water to boil in a pot and add the broc- coli. Cook until tender and cool under cold water.

In a bowl, mix all of the ingredients together and

serve on a plate!

Ingredients (1 portion)

40g arugula

1/2 tomato

5-6 slices cucumber

slices prosciutto (20g)

broccoli florets (50g)

1serving Basil Vinaigrette

14. Fluffy Omelette & Veggies

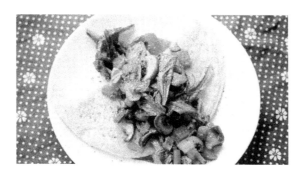

263 calories 19.29g fat8.56g carbs2.4g fiber5.26g sugar14.98g protein

Crack the eggs open in a bowl and beat with a hand mixer for 3 minutes.

Add 1tsp of olive oil to a non-stick pan and pour the whipped eggs in. Cover and cook on low heat for about 2 minutes, or until the eggs are cooked through. This will be a fluffy omelette. Fold in half and slide onto a plate.

Dice the red pepper, slice the mushrooms and chop the swiss chard. Heat the oil in a non-stick frying pan and add the red peppers. Cook for a minute, add the mushrooms and swiss chard and cook until wilted. Sprinkle the salt, pepper and garlic powder. Place over the folded omelette.

Ingredients (1 portion)

1/2 red pepper 30g swiss chard 3 mushrooms

tsp olive oil

pinch salt, pepper, garlic powder

eggs

1tsp olive oil

15. Fluffy Omelette & Veggies

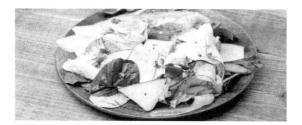

296 calories 25.93g fat9.16g carbs2.3g fiber3.53g sugar9.05g protein

Using a cabbage shredder, thinly slice the zucchini and cucumber.

Chop the spinach and cut the egg in 4.

Place everything on a plate and pour the dressing over.

Ingredients (1 portion)

1/2 zucchini (100g) 1/2 small cucumber 1/2 cup fresh spinach 1hard-boiled egg

1serving basil vinaigrette

16. Roasted Chicken Leg & Veggies

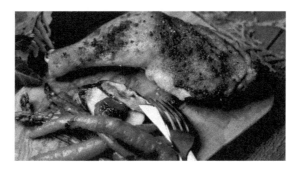

632 calories 37.78g fat9.06g carbs3g fiber4.69g sugar61.15g protein

Ingredients (2 portions)

Preheat the oven to 200C/400F.

Cut the stems off the asparagus. Slice the zucchini into vertical slices. Slice the mini carrots in half.

Place all of the veggies in a 10" cast iron skillet. Cover with the two chicken legs. Pour the olive oil over everything. Sprinkle the spices over both of the chicken legs.

Place the skillet in the oven and bake for 50 min- utes uncovered.

Take out and enjoy. Keep half for another meal.

6 asparagus spears (40g)

1/2 zucchini

100g mini carrots

2 chicken legs (600g) 1tbsp olive oil

6 cherry tomatoes (80g)

1/4 tsp salt, black pepper, cumin, paprika, chili powder

17. Grilled Veggies & FluffyOmelette

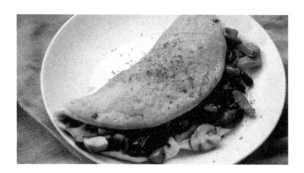

492 calories 42.26g fat8.37g carbs2.2g fiber5.38g sugar21.16g protein

Crack the eggs open in a bowl and beat with a hand

mixer for 3 minutes.

Dice the red pepper, slice the mushrooms and slice the mushrooms. Heat 1tbsp of olive oil in a non-

stick frying pan and add the red peppers. Cook for a minute, add the mushrooms and spinach and cook until wilted. Sprinkle the salt, pepper and

garlic powder. Set aside.

Add 1tbsp of olive oil to a non-stick pan and pour the whipped eggs in. Cover and cook on low heat for about 2 minutes, or until the eggs are cooked through. This will be a fluffy omelette. Place the cooked veggies on one side of the omelette and fold in half. Carefully slide onto a plate.

Ingredients (1 portion) 1/2 red pepper

1/2 cup fresh spinach 3 mushrooms

2 tbsp olive oil

pinch salt, pepper, garlic powder 3 eggs

18. **Roasted Chicken Leg & Veggies**

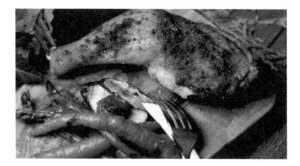

632 calories 37.78g fat9.06g carbs3g fiber4.69g sugar61.15g protein

Ingredients (2 portions)

1. Leftovers from Day 11's dinner.

Leftovers from Day 11's Dinner.

19. **Cauliflower & Veggie Ranch Salad**

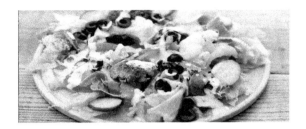

310 calories 23.22g fat12.32g carbs 4.76g fiber4.7g sugar14.90g protein

Ingredients (1 portion)

Put some water to boil in a pot and add the cauli-flower and broccoli in. Cook until tender.

Cut the tomato and slice the cucumber.

Mix the dressing ingredients together.

Add all of the salad ingredients on a plate and drizzle the dressing over.

4 lettuce leaves

3 broccoli florets (50g)

3 cauliflower florets (50g) 40g prosciutto

1/2 tomato

1/4 cup sliced cucumber

2 tbsp sliced black olives

Spicy Ranch Dressing:

1.5 tbsp mayo

1tsp unsweetened almond milk

1/4 tsp paprika powder

1/4 tsp chili oil

1/4 tsp salt, pepper

20. **Veggie Omelette**

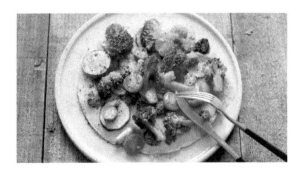

399 calories 27.97g fat9.34g carbs3.2g fiber4.42g sugar26.59g protein

Slice the broccoli, sausages, mushrooms, zucchini and cherry tomatoes in a few pieces.

Heat the oil in a medium skillet, and fry the sau- sage, mushrooms and zucchini slices for 2-3 min- utes until cooked through. Put aside.

Put some water to boil and boil the sliced broccoli and okra for 2 mintues. Take out of the boiling wa- ter, and slice the okra in 6-8 pieces.

Crack the eggs into a bowl and whisk for a minute with a whisk. Pour the egg batter in a frying pan and cook on low heat. Top with all of the veggies and meat, cover and cook until the eggs are cooked through. The omelette should just slide out of the fry- ing pan onto a plate.

Ingredients (1 portion)

eggs

broccoli (40g)

okra (10g)

mushrooms (20g) 3breakfast sausage (80g) 1/4 zucchini (50g)

4cherry tomatoes 1tsp olive oil

pinch salt & pepper

21. Kale Beef & Veggie Caesar Wrap

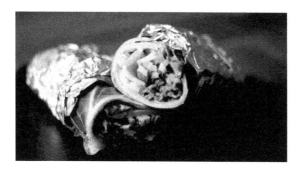

714 calories59.64g fat17.23g carbs 8.6g fiber2.66g sugar30.93g protein

Carefully trim the stem of the kale leaf so that you

can roll the leaf to make a sandwich.

Slice the avocado, red onion and tomato.

Heat the olive oil in a skillet and add the sliced beef. Sprinkle the salt, pepper and garlic powder and cook until cooked through, 1-2 minutes.

Spoon the caesar dressing over the entire leaf. On one end, add all of the toppings and carefully roll the leaf into a wrap. You can use aluminum foil to keep it from rolling out.

Ingredients (1 portion) 1portion caesar dressing 1large kale leaf (50g)

1/2 avocado 1/2 tomato 1/8 red onion

100g thinly sliced beef 1tbsp olive oil

1/4 tsp salt, pepper, garlic powder

22. Grilled Rosemary Chicken withVeggies

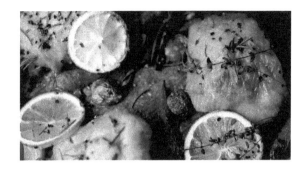

666 calories 38.08g fat7.76g carbs2.2g fiber2.38g sugar34.86g protein

Preheat the oven to 190C/410F.

Slice the radishes in half, cut the lemon into 6 slic- es, slice the red onion and cut the chicken thighs into two.

Place the chicken thighs on a baking tray that's

been covered with parchment paper (to avoid a

mess) and scatter the veggies everywhere around the thighs. Place the lemon slices over the chicken, drizzle the whole tray with the olive oil and sprinkle the salt, pep- per, rosemary and thyme over every- thing.

Place in oven and bake for 45 minutes. Take out of the oven and serve hot!

Ingredients (3 portions)

boneless chicken legs (800g) 14 mini carrots

6 garlic cloves

10 radishes 1/4 red onion 1 lemon

1tbsp rosemary 1tbsp thyme 1/2 tsp salt

1/2 tsp black pepper

2 tbsp olive oil

23. Eggs in MiniSkillet

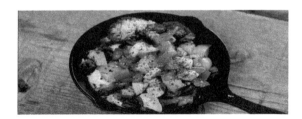

491 calories 40.87g fat15.07g carbs 8.7g fiber3.90g sugar19.34g protein

Ingredients (2 portions)

Fry the bacon until crispy in a 6" mini skillet. Chop into bits. Dice the tomato and av- ocado. Slice the okra into a few pieces.

In the same mini skillet, rack the eggs open into the bacon grease, cover and cook on low heat until cooked through. Top with the bacon bits, tomato, avocado, okra and broccoli. Sprinkle the salt, pepper and parsley over.

2 slices bacon

eggs

1/2 avocado 1 okra

1/2 tomato

3boiled broccoli (50g)

sprinkle salt, pepper, parsley

24. Grilled Rosemary Chicken withVeggies

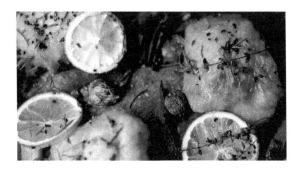

666 calories 38.08g fat7.76g carbs2.2g fiber2.38g sugar34.86g protein

1. Heat up 1/3 of the leftovers from Day 13's dinner.Ingredients (3 portions)

leftover's from Day 13's dinner

25. Grilled Chicken & Guacamole

677 calories 51.53g fat14.38g carbs 8.6g fiber2.83g sugar41.14g protein

Sprinkle the salt and pepper over the chicken thigh on both sides.

Heat the olive oil in a cast iron skillet and place the thigh skin side down. Grill on both sides until cooked through, about 4-5 minutes.

Dice the tomato and red onion. Mince the garlic and green onion. Mash the avocado and mix with the rest, and add the salt and pepper. Top over chicken along with the broccoli.

Ingredients (1 portion) 1chicken thigh with skin(150g) 1tbsp olive oil

1/2 tsp salt, pepper

1/2 avocado

1/4 tomato

1green onion stem 1slice red onion pinch salt and pepper

boiled broccoli (25g)

WEEK 3

1. WEEK 3 MENU

	Breakfast	Lunch	Dinner	Nutritional Info
Day 15	Broccoli, Bacon & Poached Egg	Grilled Rosemary Chicken with Veggies Leftovers	Spicy Chicken & Kale Salad	1450 calories 91.88g fat 19.28g net carbs 8.4g sugars 89.73g protein
Day 16	Breakfast Egg Burrito	Spicy Chicken & Kale Salad Leftovers	Chicken Meatballs & Zoodles	1386 calories 98.37g fat 15.81g net carbs 13.24g sugars 88.56 protein
Day 17	Asparagus, Bacon & Poached Egg	Spicy Chicken & Kale Salad Leftovers	Cauli Mash & Chicken Meatballs	1165 calories 75.97g fat 21.19g net carbs 11.61g sugars 86.75g protein
Day 18	Bacon, Spinach & Eggs	Chicken Meatball Lettuce Cups	Chili Con Carne & Veggies	1318 calories 97.49g fat 19.2g net carbs 11.39g sugars 79.86g protein

Day 19	Bacon, Eggs & Asparagus	Chicken Meat-ball Lettuce Cups	Cauli Mash, Green Beans & Parsley Salmon	1376 calories 95.34g fat 19.19g net carbs 19.66g sugars 96.29g protein
Day 20	Chicken Meat-balls & Eggs	Chili Con Carne	Grilled Salmon, Radishes & Green Beans	1277calories 85.05g fat 21.92g net carbs 12.96g sugars 97.14g protein
Day 21 60	Bacon, Spinach, Egg & Avocado	Chicken Meat-balls & Arugula Salad	Chili Con Carne & Veggies + Egg	1376 calories 108.15g fat 20.34g net carbs 12.32g sugars 70.24g protein

2.   WEEK 3 GROCERY LIST

Baking
Blanched Almond Flour [70g]

Canned Goods
Diced Tomato Can [500 ml]
Tomato Paste [7 ml]

Condiments
Dijon Mustard [15ml]
Lemon Juice [25 ml]
Mayonnaise [40 ml]
White Vinegar [32 ml]

Dairy
Almond Milk Unsweetened [30 ml]

Egg [12]

Meat
Bacon [18 slices]
Chicken Breast [1] {285g} withskin
Ground Beef [200g]
Ground Chicken [650g]

Oil
Chili Oil [1/4 tsp] or cayenne pepper
Olive Oil [120 ml]

Seafood & Fish
Salmon Fillet [2] {300g}
Spices
Black Pepper
Chili Powder
Cumin Powder
Dill
Garlic Powder
Himalayan Salt
Onion Powder
Oregano
Paprika Powder
Parlsey
Rosemary
Sage
Thyme

Vegetables
Arugula [40g]
Asparagus [10 stems]{200g}
Avocado [3 hass]
Basil Leaves [10 leaves]
Black Olives [1 tbsp]
Broccoli [2 heads]
Brown Mushrooms [5]
Carrot [1/4]
Cauliflower [1 head]{300g}
Celery [1/2 stick]

Cherry Tomatoes [8 cherries]

Garlic [7 cloves]

Green Beans [150g]

Kale [6 leaves]{120g}

Lettuce [9 leaves]

Okra [2]

Onion [3/4]

Parsley [4 stems]

Radishes [5]

Red Cabbage [1/8]

Shiitake Mushrooms [3]

Spinach [1 cup]

Tomato [2]

Zucchini [1 1/2]

3.   WEEK 3

Day 15 - Breakfast

1.   Broccoli, Bacon & Poached Egg

378 calories 26.48g fat   11.46g carbs 4.6g fiber   2.76g sugar   23.99g protein

Put the broccoli to boil in a pot of water and cook until tender. Take the broccoli out and place on a plate.

In a different pot, add some water and the white vinegar and put to simmer. Add the egg in a bowl. Swirl the water with a spatula and add the egg in the middle of the whirlpool. Cover and turn off the heat and cook the egg for 6 minutes exactly. Care- fully take it out and place over the broccoli.

Fry the bacon in a skillet until crispy. Chop it up into a few pieces and place over the broccoli. Driz- zle the sesame dressing over everything. Sprinkle the salt, pepper and pars- ley.

Ingredients (1 portion)

1 egg

140g broccoli (1/3 head)

3 slices bacon (36g cooked) 1portion sesame dressing 1tbsp white vinegar

pinch salt, pepper, parsley

2. *Grilled Rosemary Chicken withVeggies*

666 calories 38.08g fat   7.76g carbs   2.2g fiber   2.38g sugar   34.86g protein

1. Reheat 1/3 of the leftovers from Day 14's dinner.   Ingredients (3 portions)

1/3 leftover from day 14's dinner.

3. *Spicy Chicken & KaleSalad*

406 calories 27.32g fat   9.96g carbs   3.1g fiber   3.26g sugar   30.88g protein

Slice the chicken breast in half lenght ways. Sprinkle the salt, pepper, paprika, cumin, garlic and oregano over the chicken breasts. Heat the 1tsp of olive oil on a grill or use a

Ingredients (3 portions) 1chicken breast (285g)

1/4 tsp salt, black pepper,

Spicy Salad Dressing: 2 tbsp mayo

1tbsp lemon juice

bbq, and grill your chicken 4-5 minutes until

cooked through. Slice in 5-6 pieces.

paprika, cumin, garlic pow-   1tbsp olive oil

Slice lenghtways the zucchini. Heat the 1 tbsp of olive oil in a non-stick frying pan and add

der

1tsp oregano

1/2 tsp vinegar

1/2 tsp paprika powder

the zucchini slices. Sprinkle the salt and pep- 2 tsp olive oil

per over and grill on both sides until browned.

1/8 tsp salt

Boil the broccoli and okras for 2 minutes. Us-

small kale leaves (120g)

1/4 tsp garlic powder

ing a cabbage shredder, shred the red cab-

bage and thinly slice the watermelon radish.

6-7 broccoli with stem (100g)1 tsp oregano

Shred with your hands the kale.

In a small bowl, combine the salad dressing

ingredients.

On a large plate, cover with the kale, the rest of the veggies, and grilled chicken. Pour 1/3 of the spicy dressing over ONE portion.

Place the rest in some tupperwares for the

64 next 2 meals and keep the dressing separated

2 okra (20g)

100g red cabbage (1/8) 8 cherry tomatoes (65g) 4-5 radishes

1/2 zucchini (70g) 1tbsp olive oil

1/4 tsp hili oil or cay- enne pepper

4.   *Breakfast Egg Burrito*

538 calories 46.85g fat 10.35g carbs 6.9g fiber   1.96g sugar   20.7g protein

In a Japanese rectangular tamagoyaki frying pan, heat 1/2 tsp of olive oil. In a small bowl, whisk the two eggs together for 20 seconds or so. Pour half of the eggs into the pan, spread out evenly and cook on medium-low heat until the egg is cooked through. Carefully slide onto a plate. Repeat this step with the leftover egg mixture.

Fry the bacon until crispy.

Slice the avocado in a few slices. Slice the tomato in two. Chop the lettuce.

On each egg omelette, spread 1/2 tbsp of mayo. Cover with the lettuce, tomato, avocado and bacon and carefully roll up like a burrito.

Ingredients (1 portion)

eggs

1tsp olive oil 2 slices bacon 1lettuce leaf 1/2 avocado

1slice tomato 1tbsp mayo

5.   *Spicy Chicken & KaleSalad*

406 calories 27.32g fat   9.96g carbs   3.1g fiber   3.26g sugar   30.88g protein

Drizzle 1/2 of the dressing over 1/2 of the left- Ingredients (3 portions)

overs from day 15's dinner and enjoy!

Spicy Salad Dressing:

leftover from day 15's dinner leftover from day 15's

dinner.

6. Chicken & Herbs Meatballs

442 calories 28.34g fat   6.47g carbs   2.2g fiber   1.64g sugar   40.12g protein

Preheat the oven to 200C/400F.

Mince the garlic, shiitake and onion.

Add the olive oil to a frying pan and fry the mush- rooms, onions and garlic until tender. Turn off heat and transfer to a bowl.

Mix all of the remaining ingredients into a large

bowl and mix until well incorporated.

Place a parchment paper over a baking tray. Make 12 large meatballs and place them on the baking tray carefully making space between each meatball. The mixture is a bit sticky, but that's fine. It'll cook perfectly in the oven.

Add to the oven and cook for 25 minutes. Take out and let cool before keeping them in the fridge.

Ingredients (6 portions)

shiitake mushrooms (60g) 1/2 white onion (90g)

2 garlic cloves 1tsp olive oil

650g ground chicken

2-3 stems chopped parsley (8g)

10 leaves chopped basil (5g)

1tsp thyme, sage

1/2 tsp onion powder, salt, pepper

1/4 tsp garlic powder

1 egg

70g blanched almond flour

7. Chicken Meatballs & Zoodles

423 calories 24.2g fat 17.6g carbs   12.1g fiber

Spiralize your zucchini. Cut the meatballs into 8.

Add the tomatoes, water and spices to a pot and simmer for 5-10 minutes until desired thickness. Add the meat to the tomato sauce, mix well

Add the zoodles to the sauce and cook for a minute

or so just to get them warmed up.

8.02g sugar   36.98g protein

Ingredients (1 portion)

2 chicken meatballs

zucchini

1/2 cup diced tomato can

1/2 cup water

1/4 tsp garlic powder, onion power, basil, parsley, oregano

8. Asparagus, Bacon & Poached Egg

288 calories 21.07g fat 6.65g carbs 3.15g fiber 2.64g sugar 18.21g protein

Add some water to a small pot and the white vine- gar and put to simmer. Add the egg in a bowl. Swirl the water with a spatula and add the egg inside the middle of the whirlpool. Turn off the heat and cook the egg for 6 minutes exactly. Carefully take it out.

Fry the bacon until crispy. Cut the stems off the asparagus and fry into the bacon grease.

Place the asparagus onto a plate, cover with the bacon and poached egg and spoon the sesame dressing over. Add a bit of parlsey over everything.

Ingredients (1 portion)

6 asparagus

3 slices bacon

1 egg

1tbsp sesame dressing 1tbsp white vinegar pinch parsley

9. Spicy Chicken & KaleSalad

406 calories 27.32g fat 9.96g carbs 3.1g fiber 3.26g sugar 30.88g protein

Drizzle 1/2 of the dressing over 1/2 of the left- Ingredients (3 portions) Spicy Salad Dressing:

overs from day 15's dinner and enjoy!

leftover from day 15's dinner leftover from day 15's dinner.

10. Cauli Mash & ChickenMeatballs

471 calories 27.81g fat 18.45g carbs 7.46g fiber

Mince the garlic cloves.

Separate the cauliflower florets. Put some water to boil in a large pot and cover with a metal steamer. Add the cauliflower, cover, and cook for 5-7 minutes until tender. Once tender, transfer to a small bowl, add half the garlic, almond milk, garlic powder, onion powder, 1/2 tsp of salt and pepper. Using a

stick blender (or a food processor), puree the cauli-

flower until desired consistency.

Put the green beans to a boil and cook for 5-6 min- utes. Take out of the water into a frying pan along with the olive oil and add the leftover minced gar- lic. Sprinkle the 1/4 tsp of salt and pepper over and cook in the frying pan until the garlic gets crispy.

Reheat two chicken meatballs and place on a plate with half the cauliflower mash and half the green beans. Add the parsley over the cauli mash. Keep the other half for tomorrow.

5.71g sugar   37.66g protein

Ingredients (1 portion)

chicken meatballs

Ingredients (2 portions) 1small cauliflower (300g) 3 garlic cloves

100g green beans

1/4 tsp salt

2tbsp unsweetened almond milk 2 tsp olive oil

1/4 tsp garlic powder, onion pow-

der

1/2 tsp salt, pepper pinch parsley

11. *Bacon, Spinach & Eggs*

354 calories 25.52g fat   2.39g carbs   0.7g fiber   0.9g sugar   27.14g protein

Fry the bacon until crispy.

Chop the spinach and add to the frying pan where the bacon was. Cook in the bacon grease until wilted. Crack the eggs open over the spinach, cover and cook for 2-3 minutes until the whites are fully cooked.

Sprinkle the salt and pepper over the eggs. Slide down onto a plate with the bacon.

Ingredients (1 portion)

slices bacon (40g cooked) 2 eggs

30g spinach

pinch salt, pepper

12. Chicken Meatball Lettuce Cups

599 calories 44.65g fat   17.04g carbs 9.6g fiber   3.73g sugar   36.57g protein

Dice the tomato and avocado. Cut the meatballs into four pieces. Place two lettuce leaves on top of each other.

Mix the mayo and dijon in a small bowl. Spread half on each cup.

Add half the meatballs, tomato and avocado to

each lettuce cup. Add a bit of chopped parsley over everything.

Ingredients (1 portion)

lettuce leaves

2 chicken meatballs 1/4 tomato

1/2 avocado 1/2 tbsp mayo 1/2 tbsp dijon

pinch of parsley

13. Chili Con Carne

281 calories 19.91g fat

g carbs 3.6g fiber   5.9g sugar   14.97g protein

Ingredients (3 portions)

Dice the onion, celery and carrot. Slice the mush-

rooms. Mince the garlic.

Add the olive oil to a large pot and add all of the

veggies. Cook for 3-4 minutes until tender. Add the ground beef and cook until browned. Add the rest of the ingredients and mix to combine. Put on low

heat and simmer for 10-15 minutes until desired thickness.

74

1/4 small white onion (35)

1/2 celery stick (5g) 50g brown mushrooms 1/4 carrot (50g)

1garlic clove

tbsp olive oil

200g ground beef

1.5 cups diced tomato can (400g)

1/2 cup water

1tbsp chili powder

1/2 tbsp oregano, tomato paste 3/4 tsp cumin ground

1/2 tsp thyme

1/4 tsp salt, pepper

1/8 tsp cayenne pepper, garlic pow-

der, onion powder

14. Chili Con Carne & Veggies

365 calories 27.32g fat   17.47g carbs 7.2gfiber 6.76g sugar   16.15g protein
Ingredients (1 portion)
Top 1/3 of the chili with sliced avocado and diced tomato. Enjoy!
1/3 portion chili 1/4 avocado 1slice tomato

15. Bacon, Eggs &Asparagus

370 calories 27.90g fat   8.3g carbs   5.1g fiber
Cut the stems off the asparagus. Slice the avocado. Put some water to boil in a pot and add the aspara- gus. Cook until tender.

Fry the bacon in a skillet until crispy.

Crack the egg in the bacon grease and cook it until ready.

Add everything to the plate and sprinkle some salt and pepper over everything.

2.21g sugar   22.75g protein

Ingredients (1 portion) 1/4 avocado

bacon slices

asparagus

1 egg

pinch salt and pepper

16. Chicken Meatball Lettuce Cups

599 calories 44.65g fat   17.04g carbs 9.6g fiber   3.73g sugar   36.57g protein
Dice the tomato and avocado. Cut the meatballs into four pieces. Place two lettuce leaves on top of each other.

Mix the mayo and dijon in a small bowl. Spread half
on each cup.

Add half the meatballs, tomato and avocado to

each lettuce cup. Add a bit of chopped parsley over everything.

Ingredients (1 portion)

4 lettuce leaves

2 chicken meatballs 1/4 tomato

1/2 avocado 1/2 tbsp mayo 1/2 tbsp dijon

pinch of parsley

17. Cauli Mash, Green Beans & Parsley Salmon

407 calories 22.79g fat   14.48g carbs 5.93g fiber   4.72g sugar   36.97g protein

Reheat the cauli mash and green beans.

Mince the parsley sprig.

Rub the salmon filet with the olive oil, salt, pepper,

and parlsey.

Carefully place in a non-stick frying pan and cook on both sides for 2-3 minutes until perfectly cooked through. Once cooked, add the lemon juice over the salmon and serve with the veggies.

Ingredients (1 portion)

cauli mash leftovers from day 17 dinner

green beans leftovers from day 17

dinner

150g salmon filet 1sprig parsley 1tsp lemon juice 1tsp olive oil pinch salt, pepper

18. Chicken Meatballs & Eggs

581 calories 38.34g fat   11.48g carbs 3.7g fiber   4.33g sugar   47.87g protein

Put some water to boil in a small pot and add the broccoli. Cook until tender and add to a plate with the cherry tomatoes. Reheat the chicken meatballs and add to the plate.

Heat the olive oil in a frying pan and scramble the eggs until perfectly cooked. Sprinkle some salt and pepper over.

Ingredients (1 portion)

2 chicken meatballs

eggs

broccoli (50g)

3 cherry tomatoes 1tsp olive oil pinch salt, pepper

19. Chili Con Carne

281 calories 19.91g fat 12.4g carbs   3.6g fiber   5.9g sugar   14.97g protein

1. Reheat 1/3 of the chili and enjoy!

Ingredients (1 portion)
1/3 portion chili

20. Grilled Salmon, Radishes & Green Beans

415 calories 26.8g fat 9.04g carbs   3.7g fiber   2.73g sugar   34.3g protein

Rub the salmon with the oil, dill, salt and pepper.

Carefully place in a non-stick frying pan and cook on both sides for 2-3 minutes until perfectly cooked through. Once cooked, add the lemon juice over the salmon.

Mince the garlic clove. Put the green beans to a boil and cook for 5-6 minutes. Take out of the water into a frying pan along with the olive oil and add the minced garlic. Sprinkle the salt and pepper over and cook in the frying pan until the garlic gets crispy.

Heat the olive oil in a frying pan, add the radishes and the rosemary. Cook for 4-5 minutes until crispy. Sprinkle the salt and pepper.

Serve everything together on a plate and enjoy.

Ingredients (1 portion)

150g salmon fillet

1tsp olive oil

1/4 tsp dill, salt, black pepper

1tsp lemon juice

5 radishes (85g) 1tsp olive oil 1tbsp rosemary

pinch salt, pepper, garlic powder

50g green beans 1garlic clove

2 tsp olive oil

21. Bacon, Spinach, Egg &Avocado

347 calories 31.54g fat   5.76g carbs   4.1g fiber   0.84g sugar   11.51g protein

Fry the bacon in a skillet until crispy.

Add the spinach in the same skillet and cook in the bacon grease until wilted, and then transfer to a plate. Crack the egg in the bacon grease and cook until the white is cooked.

Slice the avocado. Put everything on a plate and sprinkle some salt and pepper over everything.

Ingredients (1 portion)

3 slices bacon

1 egg

30g spinach 1/4 avocado

pinch salt, pepper

22. Chicken Meatballs & ArugulaSalad

587 calories 44.01g fat   14.45g carbs 6.6g fiber

1. Slice the avocado, tomato and chicken meatballs. Put everything on a plate and drizzle the caesar dressing over everything.

4.16g sugar   36.32g protein

Ingredients (1 portion)

2 chicken meatballs

40g arugula

1tbsp sliced black olives 1/4 avocado

1/2 tomato

1serving caesar dressing

23. Chili Con Carne & Veggies +Egg

442 calories 32.6g fat 18.03g carbs 7.2g fiber   7.32g sugar   22.41g protein

Top 1/3 of the chili with sliced avocado, diced to- mato and sliced hard boiled egg. Enjoy!

Ingredients (1 portion)

1/3 portion chili 1/4 avocado 1slice tomato 1hard boiled egg

4. CONCLUSION

W

hether you have met your weight loss goals, you cannot just suddenly start consuming carbs again for it will shock your system. Have an idea of what you want to allow back into your consumption slowly. Be familiar with portion sizes and stick to that amount of carbs for the first few times you eat post-keto.

Start with non-processed carbs like whole grain, beans, and fruits. Start slow and see how your body responds before resolving to add carbs one meal at a time.

The things to watch out for when coming off keto are weight gain, bloating, more energy, and feeling hungry. The weight gain is nothing to freak out over; perhaps, you might not even gain any. It all depends on your diet, how your body processes carbs, and, of course, water weight. The length of your keto diet is a significant factor in how much weight you have lost, which is caused by the reduction of carbs. The bloating will occur because of the reintroduction of fibrous foods and your body getting used to digesting them again. The bloating van lasts for a few days to a few weeks. You will feel like you have more energy because carbs break down into glucose, which is the body's primary source of fuel. You may also notice better brain function and the ability to work out more.

The ketogenic diet is the ultimate tool you can use to plan your future. Can you picture being more involved, more productive and efficient, and more relaxed and energetic? That future is possible for you, and it does not have to be a complicated process to achieve that vision. You can choose right now to be healthier and slimmer and more fulfilled tomorrow. It is possible with the ketogenic diet.

This is not a fancy diet that promises falsehoods of miracle weight loss. This diet is proven by years of science and research, which benefits not only your waistline, but your heart, skin, brain, and organs. It does not just improve your physical health but your mental and emotional health as well. This diet improves your health holistically.

Keto diet provides long term health benefits compare to other diet plans. During keto diet near about 75 to 90 percent of calories comes from fats, an adequate number of calories 5 to 20 percent comes from proteins and 5 percent of calories from carb intake.

What began as a simple spark of curiosity ended on a high note: keto, a term you constantly read and heard about. Now you have all the knowledge in the world to lead a lifestyle that is truly worthy of your time, energy, and effort.

Being 50 years old or more is not bad. It is how we handle ourselves in this age that matters. Most of us would have just moved on and dealt with things as they would have arrived. That is no longer the case. It is quite literally survival of the fittest.

Do not give up now as there will be quite a few days where you may think to yourself, "Why am I doing this?" and to answer that, simply focus on the goals you wish to achieve.

A good diet enriched with all the proper nutrients is our best shot of achieving an active metabolism and efficient lifestyle. A lot of people think that the Keto diet is simply for people who are interested in losing weight. You will find that it is quite the opposite. There are intense keto diets where only 5 percent of the diet comes from carbs, 20 percent is from protein, and 75 percent is from fat. But even a modified version of this which involves consciously choosing foods low in carbohydrate and high in healthy fats is good enough.

Thanks for reading this book. I hope it has provided you with enough insight to get you going. Don't put off getting started. The sooner you begin this diet, the sooner you'll start to notice an improvement in your health and well-being.

CHAPTER

123

CONCLUSION

Whether you have met your weight loss goals, you cannot just suddenly start consuming carbs again for it will shock your system. Have an idea of what you want to allow back into your consumption slowly. Be familiar with portion sizes and stick to that amount of carbs for the first few times you eat post-keto.

Start with non-processed carbs like whole grain, beans, and fruits. Start slow and see how your body responds before resolving to add carbs one meal at a time.

The things to watch out for when coming off keto are weight gain, bloating, more energy, and feeling hungry. The weight gain is nothing to freak out over; perhaps, you might not even gain any. It all depends on your diet, how your body processes carbs, and, of course, water weight. The length of your keto diet is a significant factor in how much weight you have lost, which is caused by the reduction of carbs. The bloating will occur because of the reintroduction of fibrous foods and your body getting used to digesting them again. The bloating van lasts for a few days to a few weeks. You will feel like you have more energy because carbs break down into glucose, which is the body's primary source of fuel. You may also notice better brain function and the ability to work out more.

The ketogenic diet is the ultimate tool you can use to plan your future. Can you picture being more involved, more productive and efficient, and more relaxed and energetic? That future is possible for you, and it does not have to be a complicated process to achieve that vision. You can choose right now to be healthier and slimmer and more fulfilled tomorrow. It is possible with the ketogenic diet.

This is not a fancy diet that promises falsehoods of miracle weight loss. This diet is proven by years of science and research, which benefits not only your waistline, but your heart, skin, brain, and organs. It does not just improve your physical health but your mental and emotional health as well. This diet improves your health holistically.

Keto diet provides long term health benefits compare to other diet plans. During keto diet near about 75 to 90 percent of calories comes from fats, an adequate number of calories 5 to 20 percent comes from proteins and 5 percent of calories from carb intake.

What began as a simple spark of curiosity ended on a high note: keto, a term you constantly read and heard about. Now you have all the knowledge in the world to lead a lifestyle that is truly worthy of your time, energy, and effort.

Being 50 years old or more is not bad. It is how we handle ourselves in this age that matters. Most of us would have just moved on and dealt with things as they would have arrived. That is no longer the case. It is quite literally survival of the fittest.

Do not give up now as there will be quite a few days where you may think to yourself, "Why am I doing this?" and to answer that, simply focus on the goals you wish to achieve.

A good diet enriched with all the proper nutrients is our best shot of achieving an active metabolism and efficient lifestyle. A lot of people think that the Keto diet is simply for people who are interested in losing weight. You will find that it is quite the opposite. There are intense keto diets where only 5 percent of the diet comes from carbs, 20 percent is from protein, and 75 percent is from fat. But even a modified version of this which involves consciously choosing foods low in carbohydrate and high in healthy fats is good enough.

Thanks for reading this book. I hope it has provided you with enough insight to get you going. Don't put off getting started. The sooner you begin this diet, the sooner you'll start to notice an improvement in your health and well-being.

CPSIA information can be obtained
at www.ICGtesting.com
Printed in the USA
BVHW011516240221
R11906900001B/R119069PG600779BVX00012B/12